Keto Bread Machine Cookbook

Easy Step-by-Step Ketogenic Baking Recipes for Delicious Homemade Bread, That Use Low-Carb and Gluten-Free Recipes for Your Family and Friends at Every Meal

Paul Baker

Table of Contents

INTRODUCTION

"If you don't make time for your wellness, you will be forced to take time for your illness."

-Joyce Sunada

Investing in your health is one of the most important things you will ever do and it's time to do just that. Unlike other short-lived fad diets that come and go; the ketogenic diet has become a popular way of life for many people. What if we told you that it holds the key to weight loss, boosting your metabolism, and feeling healthier than ever before?

A ketogenic diet fondly referred to as the keto diet, is a low-carb, high-fat diet. Wait, what? Did we really just tell you that you can eat fat to lose fat? Yes, we did. Hold on a minute, isn't fat bad; isn't it unhealthy? The answer to that is both yes and no. Fat can be your friend or it can be your enemy; you just need to know how to harness the power of fat to make it work for you instead of against you. That is what the keto diet is all about learning to retrain your body to burn fat for fuel instead of feeding it carbohydrates and giving it no motivation to burn through those unwanted pounds.

The keto diet has been tried and tested and it's a proven way of eating for weight loss and improved health. Why would there be more people following a ketogenic diet than ever before if it didn't work and yield positive results? Furthermore, medical science is backing up the principles behind the diet and why it works so well.

When you think about a low-carb diet, the first thing that usually comes to mind is cutting out bread but what if you didn't have to? Bread and bread-like foods form a normal part of life for many people; sandwiches, toast, and pizza being only a few examples. When you follow the keto diet, you don't have to give up all of those delicious foods completely. You don't even have to search far and wide for keto-friendly bread at specialty health stores. You can enjoy low-carb bread and you can even make it in the comfort of your own home. We are offering you the chance to learn just how easy and delicious keto bread is and why you need to start baking some today.

So, what exactly are we going to give you?

- Learn what the keto diet is all about and what the principles are.
- Uncover the power of macros and how to calculate them for the keto diet.
- Discover the wide range of keto-friendly foods and just how much you can include while following this diet.
- Find out what the health benefits are of following a ketogenic diet.
- We will tell you about the keto baking basics, low-carb flours, and the perfect sweeteners for the job.
- Finally, we provide you with lip-smacking, out-of-this-world keto bread recipes for a variety of bread from veggie bread and cheesy loaves to pizza crust and sugarless treats that will please your sweet tooth.

There is never a better time to invest in your health and start baking fresh, tasty, low-carb keto bread at home for yourself, your family, and your friends to enjoy. With the recipes in this book, you can enjoy home-baked bread without upsetting your keto diet on your journey to a slimmer, healthier, happier you.

So, what are you waiting for?

Keep reading to find out the keto way of having your bread and eating it too.

CHAPTER 1: THE KETO WAY OF LIFE

You've heard about it and now it's to learn all about it. The ketogenic diet is growing in popularity and offering people across the globe health and weight loss success. The key is to ditch the carbs, almost, and embrace the fat. Here's an insight into what the keto diet is and how it can work for you.

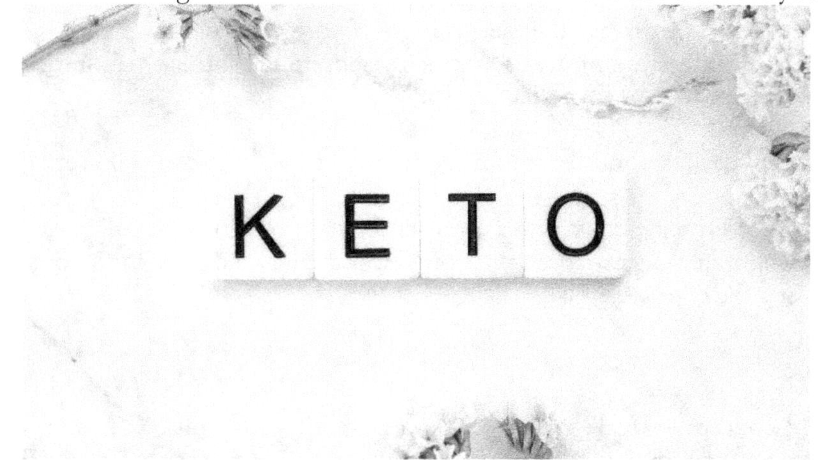

Ketogenic Diet Basics

The ketogenic diet is a lifestyle and diet buzzword that is popping up all over the place more and more often. Why? Real people are trying it, they love it, and they are seeing real results. This isn't just a celebrity dieting fad, it's the real deal and it's backed up by science. So, what is the ketogenic diet, exactly?

It is a high-fat diet with a very low carbohydrate intake. The diet is based on a macronutrient ratio of 75% fat, 20% protein, and only 5% net carbohydrates. Notice that we mention net carbs. We'll explain exactly what those are in a moment.

The idea behind the keto diet is to teach your body to burn fat for fuel instead of burning carbs as it would do while following a typical westernized diet packed with carbohydrates. A typical high-carb diet creates two byproducts, glucose and insulin. Glucose is the result of carbs being broken down into fuel; they are essentially reduced to sugars. Insulin is released by your pancreas in response to glucose entering your bloodstream once carbohydrates have been digested. It transports that glucose to the cells in your body that need energy. The problem with glucose is that it is the easiest substance to burn for fuel. If you are providing your body with constant glucose, why should it work harder to burn anything else?

The ketogenic diet gets its name from the metabolic state that it is intended to induce, ketosis. Ketosis is when your body uses fat for energy by breaking fatty acids down into ketones. The problem is that your body won't break fatty acids down into ketones for fuel when it has access to a fuel source that is much easier to burn. If you want to induce ketosis, you have to walk away from carbohydrates and embrace a diet rich in healthy fats instead.

Carbs: Ideally try to keep it to 25 grams of net carbs per day, or lower.

Protein: Protein should make up around one-quarter of your daily diet. It is an important macronutrient that provides essential nutrients for ketosis but it isn't the emphasis.

Ketogenic Diets

The concept of the ketogenic diet comes in different forms. You can follow this way of eating using a diet method that suits your needs and goals. Here are the different types of keto diets you can choose from.

Standard Ketogenic Diet
The standard ketogenic diet is the ideal starting point for beginners who are just getting into the swing of this new way of eating. It's the most basic form of the keto diet and follows the basic principles of keto such as high-fat consumption paired with protein in moderation and keeping carb intake as low as possible.

High-Protein Ketogenic Diet
A high-protein ketogenic diet is very similar to the standard keto diet except for the protein. When following a high-protein keto diet; your protein intake is increased to be as much as 35% of your diet compared to the standard keto diet's 25%.

Cyclical Ketogenic Diet
Athletes following a keto diet benefit from a cyclic ketogenic diet because carbohydrates are essential for fueling their intense workouts. A cyclic ketogenic diet offers periods of high-carb intake being alternated with low-carb intake. For instance, an athlete may follow the keto diet for five days a

week and swap to a high-carb diet, around 400 to 600 grams of carbs per day, for two days a week.

Targeted Ketogenic Diet

Active individuals who don't train as intensely and for the prolonged periods that athletes train may benefit from the targeted ketogenic diet. Here the standard keto diet is followed but with additional carbs before or after a workout. Taking in extra carbohydrates right before or after a workout helps deal with your body's energy requirements for exercise which might otherwise leave you feeling drained when following the standard ketogenic diet. Typically, you would include an extra 25 to 50 grams of carbs about 30 minutes before or after your workout.

Is a Ketogenic Diet Healthy?

Yes, the ketogenic diet is linked to several health benefits, including weight loss. Let's take a look at the reasons why the keto diet is good for your health.

Appetite

Carbs are the easiest macronutrient to digest and turn into fuel for your body. When you provide your body with food that takes longer to digest, you are less likely to feel hungry again soon after a meal or a snack. This is important when you want to lose weight and why so many traditional low-calorie diets fail. Focusing on your calorie count instead of cutting out the carbohydrate culprit while fueling up on anti-hunger foods keeps you hungry and weakens your resolve to stick to the diet.

Weight Loss

A high-fat diet for burning body fat and losing weight may seem counterintuitive but hold onto your hat because that way of thinking is about to change. Yes, you can eat fat to lose fat. When you retrain your body to burn fat from your diet as fuel, it's going to more easily and readily burn off those unwanted pounds too. The best part is that you don't have to restrict yourself to salads and a ridiculously low-calorie intake either.

Abdominal Fat

You may think that fat is fat but it's not. There are two types of excess fat. There is the fat that is under your skin and then there is fat that builds up around your internal organs in your abdomen. Excess fat collecting around your organs isn't healthy and contributes to chronic diseases such as diabetes. A low-carb diet helps reduce the amount of excess abdominal fat, reducing your risk of developing related health problems.

Energy Levels

A carb-heavy diet often sees your energy levels forming a pattern of spikes and slumps. Directly after a carb-filled meal, you are likely to experience a spike in energy as your blood sugar level spikes when carbohydrates are broken down into glucose. Not too long after that, you are likely to feel a drop in your energy levels as your pancreas releases insulin in response to a rise in your blood sugar, and glucose is removed from your bloodstream. When you swap over to a ketogenic diet, your body is burning fat for fuel which helps prevent drastic increases and decreases in blood glucose levels. Your brain is also likely to function better; thinking more clearly.

Inflammation

Inflammation happens naturally when your body is injured or sick, it's part of your immune response to that trauma or illness. However, chronic inflammation isn't natural, healthy, or fun. When your body goes into ketosis, various inflammatory pathways get turned off, reducing the severity of chronic inflammation.

Insulin Resistance and Diabetes

Insulin resistance happens when your body is constantly bombarded with high quantities of carbohydrates. Your pancreas tries to produce more and more insulin to reduce your high blood sugar levels and eventually your body becomes desensitized to all of that insulin. The result is that insulin isn't as effective anymore at lowering your blood sugar levels. Insulin resistance can often lead to the development of diabetes. When you stop overloading your body with carbs, your blood sugar levels will automatically drop and your body may become more sensitized to insulin again. Low-carb diets may help prevent the development of diabetes and insulin resistance.

The Keto Diet: What's on the Menu?

The ketogenic diet has very simple principles; eat a diet high in healthy fats, include protein in moderation, and limit carbohydrates to a minimum. The emphasis is on healthy fats. That doesn't mean greasy fried foods and saturated animal fats. Most of your fat intake should come from healthy sources such as olive oil and avocado. When you choose animal proteins, opt for grass-fed meats and fish caught in the wild.

Here's a rundown of what to include in your ketogenic diet:

Low-sugar or low-carb beverages, such as:

- Bone broth.
- Carbonated water.
- Coconut water.
- Coffee.
- Non-dairy milk.
- Select kombucha.
- Select smoothies.
- Still water.
- Still water flavored with vegetables such as cucumber.
- Tea, feel free to enjoy a variety.

Dairy products, such as:

- Grass-fed butter.
- Grass-fed ghee.
- Select cheeses.

Fats, such as:

- Avocado oil.
- Bacon fat.
- Cacao butter.

- Coconut butter.
- Coconut oil.
- Cod liver oil.
- Egg yolk.
- Grass-fed butter.
- Grass-fed ghee.
- Lard.
- Marrow and tallow.
- MCT oil (a supplement that is made from a kind of fat named medium-chain triglycerides).
- Sunflower lecithin.

Low-carb vegetables, such as:

- Asparagus.
- Avocado.
- Broccoli.
- Brussels sprouts.
- Butter greens.
- Cabbage.
- Cauliflower.
- Celery.
- Chard.
- Collards.
- Cucumbers.
- Kale.
- Kohlrabi.
- Lettuce.
- Radish.
- Spinach.
- Summer squash.
- Zucchini.

Protein, such as:

- Chicken.

- Dark meats.
- Eggs.
- Fish.
- Gelatin.
- Organ meats.
- Pork.
- Shellfish.
- Sugar-free jerky.
- Turkey.
- Whey protein concentrate.
- Wild-caught fish.

These lists of foods to include in a ketogenic diet are not even close to exhaustive but they do provide you with an idea of what you can include. It is important to be mindful of the net carb content of foods you want to include in your diet. With practice, you will be able to commit the keto-approved foods to memory and shopping for and choosing foods will become synchronized.

The Keto Diet: What's not on the Menu?

When you first start the ketogenic diet, it's a big change to make. You are going against the grain of the typical westernized diet you're accustomed to. Cutting certain foods out of your diet and avoiding them in social situations can be difficult at first. The good news is that it's not mission impossible and keto-friendly foods and meals are delicious. It is important to constantly monitor your carb intake. It is very easy to miscalculate or lose track of your carbs if you aren't paying attention and that could bring your body out of a state of ketosis, setting your progress back.

Here's a rundown of what to exclude and avoid on a ketogenic diet:

High-sugar drinks, such as:

- Beer.
- Carbonated drinks.
- High-sugar alcoholic drinks.
- High-sugar coffees.
- Juices.
- Sports drinks.

Starchy vegetables, such as:

- Carrots.
- Parsnips.
- Peas.
- Potatoes.
- Yams.

High-carb fruits, such as:

- Apples.
- Bananas.
- Grapes.
- Mangoes.
- Oranges.
- Papaya.

Beans and legumes, such as:

- Black beans.
- Black-eyed peas.
- Chickpeas.
- Kidney beans.
- Lentils.
- Pinto beans.

Grains, such as:

- Barley.
- Oats.
- Rice.
- Sorghum.
- Wheat.

Sugars, such as:

- Agave.
- Cane sugar.
- Honey.
- Maple syrup.

These lists of foods to cut out of a ketogenic diet are not even close to exhaustive but they do provide you with an idea of what you should take off the menu. It is important to be mindful of the net carb content of foods. With practice, you will be able to easily remember which foods to avoid and shopping for and choosing foods will become synched.

Keto Macros and Calculating Them

Macronutrients, or macros, are the nutrients your body needs in larger quantities than vitamins and minerals and they make up your calorie count for the day. Fat, protein, and carbohydrates are the three macronutrients.

Macronutrient quantities for the standard ketogenic diet are:

- 75% fat.
- 20% protein.
- 5% carbohydrates.

Calculating Macros

There are a few simple steps that will help you calculate your macronutrient needs on the ketogenic diet.

Calories

What is your goal?

- Weight loss (calorie deficit).
- Weight gain (calorie surplus).
- Weight maintenance (calories in equal calories out).

Your caloric needs will depend on your goal and how many calories you burn per day. To determine your daily calorie needs, you must figure out your basal metabolic rate and then multiply that by a basic number depending on your activity level. Your basal metabolic rate is the number of calories your body needs per day to keep going while in a state of rest.

Base metabolic rate calculation:

- Metric calculation for men: 66.47 + (13.75 x weight in kilograms) + (5.003 x height in centimeters) − (6.755 x age in years).
- Imperial calculation for men: 66 + (6.2 × weight in pounds) + (12.7 × height in inches) − (6.76 × age in years).
- Metric measurement for women: 655 + (9.563 × weight in kilograms) + (1.850 × height in cm) − (4.676 × age in years).
- Imperial calculation for women: 655 + (4.35 × weight in pounds) + (4.7 × height in inches) - (4.7 × age in years).

For example, using the imperial calculation for a woman of 150 pounds, 66 inches tall (5ft 6in), and 30 years old:

- 655 + (4.35 × 150) + (4.7 × 66) - (4.7 × 30).
- 655 + 625.5 + 310.2 − 141 = BMR of 1,450 calories needed per day.

Your total caloric needs to maintain your weight is made up of your BMR + calories burned based on activity level.

- A sedentary lifestyle with almost no exercise: BMR x 1.2 = daily calories.
- Lightly exercise: BMR x 1.375 = daily calories.
- Moderate exercise 3 to 5 days per week: BMR x 1.55 = daily calories.
- Very active, exercising 6 to 7 days per week: BMR x 1.725 = daily calories.
- Extra active, exercising 6 to 7 days per week plus having a physically demanding job: BMR x 1.9 = daily calories.

For example, a 30-year-old, 150 pound woman who is 66 inches tall and does moderate exercise:

BMR 1,450 x 1.55 = 2,247.5 calories per day to maintain weight.

Carbohydrates
Ketogenesis should be activated with a carb intake of 20 to 50 grams of net carbs, or less, per day. However, the precise amount may vary from person to person and your activity level. Active individuals may need additional carbs before or after a workout.

Start with 20 to 25 grams of carbs per day and if you are experiencing difficulties with that amount, increase it to up to 50 grams. You can use your daily caloric needs as a guideline for determining your carbohydrate needs. For example, if you have a calorie intake of less than 2,000 per day, 20 grams should be sufficient to reach your goal of 5% of your caloric intake coming from carbs.

Carb to calorie guideline:

- Less than 2,000 calories per day: 20 grams or less.
- 2,000 to 2,500 calories per day: 25 to 30 grams or less.
- 2,500 to 3,000 calories per day: 30 to 35 grams or less.
- More than 3,000 calories per day: 35 to 50 grams.

Carbs have approximately four calories per gram. Convert your daily carb needs into calories by multiplying the number of grams by four. For example, 20 x 4 = 80 calories per day should come from carbohydrates.

When calculating your carbohydrate needs, you count the net carbs in food, not the total carbs. Net carbs are different from total carbs in that carbohydrates can be broken down into two parts: sugars and fiber. Net carbs refer to the total amount of carbohydrates that your body can absorb from a food item. Since your body cannot digest and absorb fiber, those carbs are essentially cut out of the equation. You can calculate the net carbs of a food item by subtracting the fiber from the total carb content. For instance, if the total carbohydrate content of a food product is listed at 30 but the fiber is listed as 20; there are only 10 net carbs in that food.

Protein
You can estimate your daily protein needs by considering your fitness goal and how active you are.

- A sedentary lifestyle with not much exercise.
- A moderately active lifestyle with moderate physical exercise two days per week or more.
- A very active lifestyle with intense exercise three days a week or more.
- Daily protein needs can be calculated using a simple guideline:
- Weight maintenance or a sedentary lifestyle: 0.6 grams of protein for each pound of bodyweight.
- Weight loss or a moderately active lifestyle: 0.9 grams of protein for each pound of bodyweight.
- Weight gain, muscle gain, or a very active lifestyle: 1.1 grams of protein for each pound of bodyweight.

For example, someone who wants to lose weight leads a moderately active lifestyle and weighs 150 pounds needs 0.9 grams of protein per day multiplied by 150. 0.9 x 150 = 135 grams of protein daily.

Protein has approximately four calories per gram. Convert your daily protein needs into calories by multiplying the number of grams by four. 135 x 4 = 540 calories per day should come from protein.

Fat
Fat should make up the majority of your daily calorie intake and based on your carb and protein-calorie conversions, you can determine your fat calories by deducting carb and protein calories from your daily caloric needs.

For example:

- 2,000 calories per day required.
- 20 grams of carbs = 80 calories.
- 135 grams of protein = 540 calories.
- Calculation: 2,000 – 620 = 1,380 calories should come from fat.

Fat has approximately nine calories per gram. Convert your daily fat calories into grams by dividing the number of calories by nine. 1,380 ÷ 9 = 153.3 grams of fat daily.

Macros Percentage
You probably don't need to perform this step but it can help you confirm whether your macro percentage is correct and suitable for a standard keto diet.

Divide the number of calories for each macronutrient by your daily caloric total and then multiply that number by 100 to work out the percentage.

Carbs: 80 ÷ 2,000 = 0.04. 0.04 x 100 = 4%.

Protein: 540 ÷ 2,000 = 0.27. 0.27 x 100 = 27%.

Fat: 1,380 ÷ 2,000 – 0.69. 0.69 x 100 = 69%.

4% + 27% + 69% = 100%.

Your macro percentage doesn't have to be exact to the last 1% of your daily caloric needs, a small amount of wiggle room is allowed. However, as you can see, based on the above calculation, fat makes up nearly 70%, protein makes up just over 25%, and carbs make up just under 5% which is well in line with the 5% recommendation for the standard ketogenic diet.

Macro Meals

Once you have worked out your keto macro needs, you can work on building your meals according to the grams of fat, protein, and carbs in different foods. This requires some work to create lists of foods and their macro content. You can also work out portion sizes based on those macros in each food.

For example:
Percentage of daily calories per meal: 2,000 calories ÷ 4 meals per day = 500 calories per meal.

- Carbs per meal at 4%: 500 x 0.04 = 20 grams per meal.
- Protein per meal at 27%: 500 x 0.27 = 135 grams per meal.
- Fat per meal at 69%: 500 x 0.69 = 345 grams per meal.

CHAPTER 2: BAKING THE KETO WAY

Advantages of Home-Baked Bread

Baking your bread at home may need you to roll up your sleeves and put some elbow grease into it but making your bread definitely has its benefits. Thinking about making your bread and investing in a recipe book means that you already have the desire. Let's stoke that home-baking fire with great reasons why baking your bread in the comfort of your kitchen can be such a game-changer in your life.

Complete control

You have complete control over the ingredients that you include in your bread. You can accommodate various food allergies and dietary needs or restrictions with recipes that are gluten-free to low in sugar.

By using your kitchen as your workspace, you can avoid potential contamination by allergens, such as nuts. When dealing with allergens that could be potentially fatal, you can't be too careful and if there are no allergens present, there is no risk of contamination.

You can cut out unwanted, and potentially harmful, additives and preservatives. Fresh, home-baked bread doesn't have a long shelf-life because it is preservative-free. However, that is a small tradeoff for the health benefits of not including preservatives. The world is moving more and more toward natural foods and eating as naturally as possible because it's just so much healthier. Cutting out artificial additives and preservatives takes you one step closer to optimum health.

Added sugar and salt are everywhere. Have you ever wondered why people are cautioned about adding salt and sugar to their prepared meals when they sit down to eat them? So many food products already have added sugar and salt in them; yes, even in the bread you eat. Taking in too much salt or sugar isn't good for your health or your waistline. Home-baked bread is generally lower in salt and sugar and you can customize your recipes for even lower levels if you want to.

Baking your bread at home gives you the option to swap out traditional saturated fats for healthier fats such as olive oil. The only time homemade bread could contain unhealthy saturated fats is if you decide to include them by using ingredients like vegetable shortening. This is a great advantage if you, or someone in your family, suffers from cholesterol and/or heart problems.

Macros can be a concern for health-conscious individuals or if you are following a specific diet, such as the keto diet. Making your own bread puts you in the driver's seat. You can calculate and control the macronutrient quantities by using different recipes specifically designed for various dietary requirements.

Health

Baking your bread at home offers you the chance to enjoy the healthiest bread possible. You can use the most nutritious, whole, unprocessed ingredients when you make homemade bread. If you have to choose processed ingredients, you have the decision-making power to ensure that they are as minimally processed as possible when picking your bread ingredients. Specialty bread that contains added fruits or vegetables can be made from scratch, avoiding the use of canned or packaged ingredients.

Another perk of baking your bread at home is that it is always fresh. You can make bread as and when you need it and make small quantities so that it doesn't stand around getting stale. Who doesn't love fresh, wholesome bread for their sandwiches?

Homemade bread can help you avoid empty calories. Various bread may contain added dextrose or high-fructose corn syrup. Neither of these ingredients offers any real nutritional value and drives up the calorie count of the bread. Taking in too many calories may lead to gaining weight and developing several health complications such as fatty liver and diabetes.

Creativity and Therapy

Baking your bread at home allows you to be creative. You can make a variety of different types of bread from plain sandwich loaves to specialty loaves that contain cheese, fruits, or vegetables.

Home baking lets you experiment with it by using different types of flour. Each type of flour brings some unique qualities to the bread from subtle differences in how the bread tastes to its texture. You can test out a variety of flours and find the one that offers you just the right taste and the perfect texture so that you love every single morsel.

The whole process of baking bread can be a very therapeutic experience, especially if you love being in the kitchen. Not only can you let your creativity run wild. The repetitive motions of kneading bread can be similar to meditation, calming your mind. The effort that you put into the kneading process may also act as a stress reliever by doing something physical to work that stress out of your system.

The smell of baking bread is a happy one, filling your kitchen with the scent of a happy home, not unlike the smell of baking cookies, and can evoke fond memories from childhood or special experiences. The cherry on top with home baking is the sense of accomplishment it can bring you. Seeing, smelling, and then tasting the delicious fruits of your labor is a very fulfilling feeling which helps to boost your mood and confidence.

Who doesn't love to receive homemade treats, straight from the heart? Home-baked bread comes in all shapes, sizes, and flavors; they are the perfect gift for friends and family. Healthy, tasty bread straight from your kitchen is a gift that won't go to waste, tells people that you care, and is always a viable option, irrespective of the occasion.

Time and Money

There is a common misconception that making bread at home is a time-consuming affair. This doesn't have to be the case, especially if you make use of a bread machine. Even if you don't have a bread machine and use a traditional oven for baking bread, you can find and use recipes that won't take forever to make. Recipes vary from basic, quick bread to more complex bread that takes longer to put together. You can bake simpler bread when your schedule is busy and spend time getting creative with more complex recipes when you aren't as busy.

Not only does homemade bread not have to be a time drain, but it can also save you money. The cost of making homemade bread may well work out cheaper than you think. When you add up the cost of the ingredients and the number of bread loaves those ingredients make, you may be surprised by just how affordable it is to make a single loaf of home-baked bread.

Taste

We've saved the best for last. The delicious taste of homemade bread is reason enough to ditch the plain, often tasteless, bread you can buy in a store. Food is fuel for your body, but eating is an experience and taste is a very important part of that whole experience. It's also the taste of home, it's wholesome, and you can taste the nutritional goodness in every single bite.

Keto Baking Basics

People have been baking at home for millennia. Flatbread was around before the use of yeast in baking was discovered. Safe to say, it's not a new concept even if our modern world values instant gratification and convenience over delicious, healthy bread. Bread has evolved from its humble beginnings to the seemingly endless variety available today. Along with that, baking ingredients and equipment have evolved too. There is so much to choose from, where do you start and what do you need to begin baking bread in the comfort of your own home?

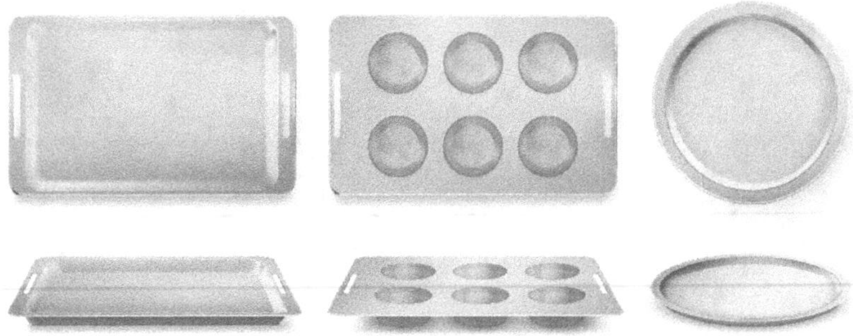

Bread-Baking Equipment

Even more varied than the different types of bread you can bake is the different bits and pieces of equipment available for baking that bread. It can be confusing to make choices and decisions. Depending on whom you listen to or which blog you read, everybody has their own opinion on what is necessary for baking bread at home. We're going to take the mystery out of home bread making for you and give you a rundown of must-have equipment you definitely need as well as some extras that aren't essential but would make your baking life easier.

Bare Necessities

When you are just beginning to bake bread, you won't need to invest in tons of equipment just yet. You can get to that later when you progress to baking a wider assortment of bread. For now, you need a few simple necessities to get you started.

Standard Loaf Pans

You cannot bake bread without loaf pans. They come in a variety of sizes from mini to large. There are also different materials to choose from like glass or metal. Should you get plain or non-stick? Well, the first step is to invest in a standard size loaf pan, or two. Metal is the most common material for a loaf pan and it's more durable than glass. Non-stick pans make getting your bread out easier and you won't have to use lots of added greasing agents to prevent sticking.

Bread Machine

The traditional way to make bread is using an oven. However, it may not be the most convenient method of baking your bread. Bread machines come in a wide range of brands and designs, each with different functions and settings. Some bread machines will help you do everything from mixing and kneading dough to baking the bread. It is important to find a bread machine that suits your needs and is easy to use.

Bread Knife

This may seem like a no-brainer but if you don't usually slice up loaves of bread, you may not have a bread knife in the kitchen. Home-baked bread doesn't come out of the bread machine or oven perfectly sliced; you are going to have to carve it up into slices yourself. A good serrated bread knife will hold up against crispy crusts without squishing your bread flat in the process; cutting each slice will be a synch.

Mixing Bowls

If you're not using a bread machine that does it all in one, you're going to need to mix and proof your dough (allow it to rise) in a mixing bowl. Have a variety of sizes on hand so that you can quickly grab the right size bowl for the amount of dough you're making.

Reusable Bowl Covers

Traditionally kitchen towels or clear plastic wrap have been used to cover the bowl while the bread is proofing. Sometimes traditional isn't the best way to go. Stop wasting plastic wrap that is only good for a single-use and opt for reusable bowl covers. They are made of cotton, they are washable, and they come in different sizes so that they perfectly fit various sizes of mixing bowls. While cotton is breathable, it will also keep moisture in, a key part of good proofing.

Digital Cooking Thermometer

When yeast is involved, the temperature is a very important aspect of baking bread. Yeast needs a warm, moist environment to work its rising magic. When adding water to the dough or to proof the yeast, the temperature is vital. If the water is too cold, the yeast won't rise. If the water is too hot, you can expect a similar outcome. A digital cooking thermometer is quick and easy to read and will take the guesswork out of achieving the perfect water temperature of 110°F.

Bread Box

Proper bread boxes do wonders for keeping your delicious homemade bread fresh. They also come in a dizzying array of colors and designs to fit perfectly in with your kitchen décor. Having a designated bread box also makes it easy to reach for your bread without having to look around for it. Remember that home-baked bread doesn't contain all the preservatives of store-bought bread and therefore has a shorter shelf-life. A bread box helps to stave off going stale for a little while longer.

Dough Whisk

While a wooden spoon works fine for mixing bread dough, a dough whisk will make your life so much easier. It may look strange when you first see one but the spaces in the whisk let you mix all the ingredients more thoroughly and aerate the mixture at the same time.

Electric Mixer Dough Hook Attachment

If you have a sturdy electric mixer, you are going to want to use it for mixing your bread dough, and for that, you're going to need a dough hook attachment. Using an electric mixer takes all the hard work out of combining the ingredients, saving you the hassle and saving you time.

Wire Cooling Rack

For bread to retain a crispy crust, it needs to breathe after baking. If you let it sweat in the loaf pan, you will end up with a softer crust. Turn your bread out onto a wire cooling rack as soon as it comes out of the oven for the best chance at achieving that super crispy crust.

Non-Essentials

Now we're getting to the bread baking equipment that's great to have but won't make or break your ability to make tasty homemade bread.

Baking Stone

Baking stones work in a similar way to baking sheets for cookies. They are useful for baking bread and bread rolls that don't need the same kind of structured baking as normal bread. What does a baking stone do that a baking sheet doesn't do? It absorbs some of the moisture from the outside of the baked bread while cooling so that a crunchy crust forms.

Mini Loaf Pan

Miniature loaf pans are brilliant for baking pint-sized loaves. Want to bake a whole batch of bread as gifts, use a miniature loaf pan. You will get several little loaves from a single bake and they make adorable gifts.

Bowl Scraper

Bread dough is notorious for being sticky. When it's not sticking to your hands, it's sticking to the inside of the mixing bowl. A silicone bowl scraper will help you tame that stickiness and scrape every last bit of dough from your bowl. The perk of a bowl scraper is that it doesn't just work for bread dough; it comes in handy for a variety of cooking and baking activities.

Bench Scraper

This tool is not essential for baking bread but it makes your baking life a breeze, it's a bench scraper. Not only can you easily scrape the dough off your working surface after kneading it, but this tool is also super versatile. You can use it as part of the kneading process as well as to section up your dough for bread rolls, braided bread, etc.

Indoor Thermometer

Bread dough rises best at a certain temperature. If the air temperature is too cold or too hot, you risk running into trouble, such as failure to rise. Yeast is added to a recipe specifically so that the bread can rise, if you wanted flatbread you could just have left the yeast out. So, you want to let your dough proof in the right conditions. An indoor thermometer will let you know whether your kitchen is the perfect combination of 75°F and 60% to 80% humidity for the ideal proofing environment.

Countertop Dough Proofer

Making your own bread is easy and fun but it can be temperamental at times. One of those times is when the temperature isn't just right for the perfect proofing. Good proofing environments are hard to come by in cooler climates, making a countertop proofer a great piece of equipment to help you achieve consistent results.

Couche Cloth

A couche cloth is an important tool for making bread such as baguettes and bread rolls that need to retain a certain shape but are not baked in a loaf pan. Some bread can be baked using a baking sheet or a baking stone but you still need to offer them support so that they maintain their shape. A couche cloth is a heavy-duty linen cloth that is used to support shaped bread during their final proof.

Low-Carb Flours and Using Them

Flour is the main ingredient in the majority of baked goodies. However, when you're on the low-carb keto diet, flour can be a big challenge. As we've explained, wheat flour is not on the menu. So, where does that leave you when you want to lay your hands on bread, cookies, cakes, etc.?

You can start baking your very own delicious bread. It's easy, it's quick, and we're going to decode the alternatives to wheat flour that you can use when following a keto diet and just how to incorporate them in recipes.

Important Aspects of Low-Carb Flour

Carbohydrates: The keto diet emphasizes low-carb foods. Using low-carb flour is therefore important. Be mindful of the carbohydrate content of the flour you choose. Another important aspect is that your flour is as minimally processed or refined as possible to offer complex carbs instead of simple carbs. Complex carbs take longer to digest, avoiding blood sugar spikes and keeps you feeling fuller for longer.

Fat: Another part of the keto diet is that it has a relatively high-fat content. Flours containing healthy fats are preferable.

Fiber: Dietary fiber is an important part of digesting complex carbs more slowly for a steady release of glucose into your bloodstream to avoid blood sugar spikes and keep you feeling fuller for longer.

Calories: Some low-carb flours are very high in calories. When you can substitute a like-for-like quantity of low-carb flour for regular wheat flour, it is important to be aware that the calorie content of the food will increase to avoid taking in too many calories.

Nutrients: Choosing flour that offers more nutrients than wheat flour gives you a better chance of meeting all of your daily nutritional needs.

Glycemic Index: The glycemic index of a food refers to how quickly or how slowly they cause your blood sugar to rise when you eat them. Being aware of the glycemic index of the flour used is especially important for diabetics. Complex carbs generally have a lower glycemic index than simple carbs.

Top Low-Carb Flour Substitutes

Cricket Flour

This flour may be as low-carb as they come but it may not appeal to everyone. The name is pretty self-explanatory, this flour is made from crushed dried crickets.

- Taste Profile: Said to be slightly nutty.
- Texture: Chewy, not 'cakey.'
- Where to get cricket flour: Online, it is not a common supermarket item.
- Substitution: You can substitute cricket flour at a ratio of 1:1 by replacing wheat flour with the same amount of cricket flour. Cricket flour can also be mixed with nut flours that have the same wheat flour to nut flour ratio such as almond flour.

Cricket Flour Benefits

- It contains an adequate amount of all nine essential amino acids, making it a whole protein.
- Cricket flour is eco-friendly.
- Cricket flour is made from insects so it's gluten-free.
- It's a rich source of nutrients such as copper, manganese, zinc, B vitamins, and iodine.
- Cricket flour is a source of healthy fatty acids.

Possible Disadvantages

- Cricket flour is made from insects which may be off-putting for some.
- Using this flour produces a less 'cakey' texture than other low-carb flour substitutes.
- Cricket flour isn't readily available and is generally only found online.

Flaxseed Flour

Flaxseed flour isn't a newcomer to the low-carb flour arena. It is widely used as a wheat flour substitute and offers several health benefits.

- Taste profile: Mildly nutty.
- Texture: Thickens and adds texture to recipes.
- Substitution: You can substitute flaxseed flour at a ratio of 1:1/3 plus add one tablespoon of either milk or water. For example, substitute one cup of wheat flour with 1/3 cup of flaxseed flour and one tablespoon of milk or water.
- Where to get flaxseed flour: health food stores, online

Flaxseed Flour Benefits

- Flaxseed is a rich source of nutrients and omega-3 fatty acids.
- It may help lower bad LDL cholesterol and improve overall cholesterol, preventing heart disease.
- It improves blood sugar levels.
- Flaxseed flour may assist with lowering blood pressure.
- It's a rich source of quality protein.
- The insoluble fiber content of flaxseed flour may help lower blood sugar levels.

Possible Disadvantages

- Flaxseed flour adds a lot of texture and greatly thickens recipes which may present a problem in baking.
- It is not recommended for women who are pregnant or breastfeeding because not enough scientific studies have been made, and the results of tests are controversial and contradictory.

- Flaxseed flour may not be readily available in supermarkets.

Lupin Flour

Lupin flour is made from sweet lupin beans that have been ground into a powder. Despite being a legume, it is surprisingly low in carbohydrates and high in fiber. It is also very high in protein. The low-carb content makes lupin flour a popular choice for those following the ketogenic diet.

- Taste profile: Bitter but the bitterness lessens when cooked or baked.
- Texture: Similar to non-keto-friendly baked foods
- Where to get lupin flour: Some supermarkets, online, homemade by blending whole sweet lupin beans in a blender
- Substitution: It's recommended to mix lupin flour with another low-carb keto-friendly flour, especially almond flour, to help dilute the bitter flavor. When mixing almond flour and lupin flour for a recipe, always use the original amount of flour required but substitute half of that amount for lupin flour. For example, if a recipe calls for 100g of almond flour, substitute 50g of lupin flour and use almond flour for the remaining 50g of flour the recipe calls for.

Lupin Flour Benefits

- It's gluten-free.
- Lupin flour can be used in a variety of cooked and baked goodies from pancakes and biscuits to bread.
- This flour has a high fiber and protein content.
- Lupin flour may be beneficial in lowering blood pressure.
- Bad LDL cholesterol levels may be lowered, helping to keep your heart healthy.

Potential Disadvantages

- Lupin is closely related to peanuts and soy. People with peanut, nut, or soy allergies may have an adverse allergic reaction to lupin flour.
- It has a naturally bitter taste which may affect food if it isn't mixed

with low-carb flour.

Macadamia Nut Flour

Macadamia nut flour is made from crushed macadamia nuts. It's extremely tasty but not as readily available as other low-carb flours.

- Taste Profile: Mildly nutty and slightly sweet.
- Texture: moist and chewy.
- Where to get macadamia nut flour: Select supermarkets and health stores, online, homemade using a blender to powder whole nuts.
- Substitution: You can substitute macadamia nut flour for wheat flour at a ratio of 1:1 by replacing the amount of wheat flour with the same amount of macadamia flour.

Macadamia Nut Flour Benefits

- Macadamia nuts are high in essential minerals and vitamins such as manganese and thiamine.
- It is a source of healthy, unsaturated fats.
- Macadamia nut flour, as with other nut flours, is packed with free-radical busting antioxidants.
- The healthy fats and nutrients found in macadamia nuts may improve heart health and lower bad LDL cholesterol levels.
- Macadamia nut flour can be mixed with other low-carb flour substitutes that also have a substitution ratio of 1:1.

Potential Disadvantages

- Macadamia nut flour is very high in calories.
- It is an expensive low-carb substitute.
- Made from nuts, macadamia flour poses an allergen risk.

Walnut Flour

Walnut flour is made from crushed walnuts. It is less common than other nut flours but offers great health benefits.

- Taste Profile: Strong walnut flavor but could be mixed with almond meal to lessen the taste.
- Texture: Moist, soft, chewy.
- Where to get walnut flour: Some supermarkets, homemade blending whole nuts in a blender, online.
- Substitution: You can substitute walnut flour at a ratio of 1:1 by replacing the amount of wheat flour with the same amount of walnut flour.

Walnut Flour Benefits

- Walnuts are a rich source of antioxidants that help tame free radicals and the damage they do to your body's cells. The antioxidants come from vitamin E, polyphenols, and melatonin found in walnut skins.
- Walnuts may help lower your bad LDL cholesterol, keeping your heart healthy.
- Part of the high-fat content of walnut flour is the presence of omega-3 fatty acids which are an essential healthy fat and must be included regularly for a healthy diet.
- Some polyphenols found in walnuts may help to reduce inflammation in your body. Inflammation is a big component of some chronic diseases such as type 2 diabetes and heart disease, and cancer.
- A suggested benefit of including walnuts in your diet is weight control. Walnuts may help with appetite control which could reduce snacking and overeating.

Possible Disadvantages

- Walnuts may trigger a nut allergy.

- It is high in calories.

Almond Meal/Flour

- Taste Profile: Nutty
- Texture: moist, soft, chewy
- Substitution: You can substitute almond meal at a ratio of 1:1 by replacing the amount of wheat flour with the same amount of almond meal.
- Where to get almond meal: Supermarkets, homemade in a blender, online

Almond Meal Benefits

- It's high in nutrients, especially copper, vitamin E, riboflavin (a B vitamin), magnesium, and manganese.
- Almond meal is a rich source of fiber and protein.
- Almond meal is made from nuts so it's gluten-free.
- Almond meal could be healthy for your heart. Almonds may help lower bad LDL cholesterol as well as total cholesterol. They may also help to decrease your blood pressure. All of these benefits are good for your ticker.

Possible Disadvantages

- While the almond meal is a super substitute for wheat flour, it is not without its potential faults. Here's what to think about when considering almond flour in baking recipes.
- The fats in almond flour are delicate and oxidation can happen when baking at high temperatures. It is advised to check recipes and use almond flour for baking at lower temperatures.
- It has a high-calorie content.
- Almonds are a nut and may trigger a nut allergy.
- The high oxalate content of almond flour could cause problems for individuals who are prone to kidney stones or if a low-oxalate diet has been prescribed.

Coconut Flour

Coconut flour is a cheaper alternative to the almond meal but it is also vastly different. Made from dried and ground coconut meat, it has a much drier texture than almond flour, meaning that much less is needed when substituting coconut flour for wheat flour in a recipe. Another difference is that coconut flour absorbs lots of liquids from a recipe, such as milk or eggs that are included.

- Taste Profile: Coconut flour lends a coconut flavor to baked goods.
- Texture: Potential to be dry if too much is used.
- Substitution: Coconut flour can be used as a wheat flour substitute at a ratio of 1:1/4. For example, one cup of wheat flour can be substituted with ¼ cup of coconut flour.
- Where to get coconut flour: Supermarkets, online.

Coconut Flour Benefits

- Coconut flour is high in nutrients, particularly copper, selenium, manganese, and magnesium.
- It's high in fiber.
- Coconut flour is low carb.
- It may offer your heart health benefits such as lowering LDL cholesterol and the level of blood triglycerides, or fat in your blood.
- A potentially beneficial ingredient found in coconut flour is monolaurin which can help boost your immune system.
- Coconut flour is gluten-free.

Possible Disadvantages

- Those who are sensitive to or intolerant of salicylates may be negatively affected by the high-salicylate content of coconut flour.
- Coconut flour has the potential to produce dry baked goods.
- Coconut flour has a higher carbohydrate content than various other low-carb flours.

Psyllium Husk Powder

Psyllium husk powder is made by grinding up the outer shell or husk of the seeds from the Plantago ovata plant. It is used for baking and for thickening food. It has a high water-soluble fiber content, absorbing liquid and offering a low net carb content of only 11.1g per 100g. This is not a full substitute for nut flour and should rather be added to the recipe separately in a small amount.

- Taste profile: Mild and oat-like.
- Texture: Moist, non-crumbly.
- Where to get psyllium husk powder: Health stores, online.
- Substitution: Psyllium husk powder cannot be substituted for nut flour but it can be added to another low-carb flour. It bulks out recipes and offers a more bread-like texture. For this purpose, add a tablespoon or two of psyllium husk powder to the low-carb flour you are using as a wheat flour substitute.

Psyllium Husk Powder Benefits

- Psyllium husk is high in water-soluble fiber.
- It is used to bulk out recipes, making you feel fuller for longer.
- Due to its bulking ability, this powder may aid in weight loss.
- It may contribute to lowering blood pressure.
- The high fiber content may help individuals with digestive problems when added to recipes.
- Psyllium husk powder may help lower bad LDL cholesterol levels.

Potential Disadvantages

Taking in too much psyllium husk powder may lead to digestive system blockage caused by too much indigestible fiber.

Low-Carb Four Nutritional Value Chart

Per 100g	Cricket Flour	Flaxseed Flour	Lupin Flour	Macadamia Flour	Walnut Flour	Almond Flour	Coconut Flour
Calories	471	534	247	718	654	571	443
Carbs	11.7g	28.9g	40.0g	14.2g	13.7g	21.4g	59.3g
Fiber	5.9g	27.3g	36.7g	8.6g	6.7g	10.7g	37.5g
Sugars	1.5g	1.5g	3.3g	4.6g	2.6g	3.6g	6.8g
Net Carbs	1.6g	1.6g	3.3g	5.6g	7.0g	10.7g	21.8g
Fat	17.6g	42.2g	6.7g	75.8g	65.2g	50.0g	15.0g
Protein	64.7g	18.3g	40.0g	7.9g	15.2g	21.4g	17.5g

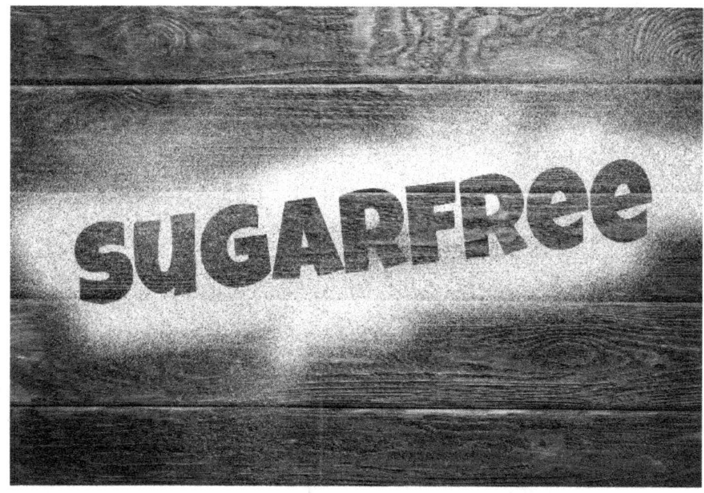

Substituting Low-Carb Flour for Wheat Flour

A pillar of the ketogenic diet is low-carb foods. While there are specific ketogenic recipes available, you can make regular baked goodies more keto-friendly by substituting the wheat flour that is called for with low-carb flour. This is especially useful when baking for a group of people who are not following a keto diet but you don't want to either be the odd one out not eating anything or completely mess up your keto diet.

It is important to experiment with low-carb flour substitutes. A general substitution guideline has been provided but you may need to do a little fine-tuning depending on the particular recipe. The suggested substitution amounts are a good starting point but you probably shouldn't put all your faith into a perfect result for a first-time test bake. Avoid substituting wheat flour with low-carb flour for the first time when making a recipe you haven't substituted before.

Different low-carb flours also bring their own taste profile to the table, literally. It will take time and experimentation to find the low-carb flour that you enjoy the most and that works the best for a variety of recipes.

Keto-Friendly Sweeteners

Carb avoidance is the name of the game when following the ketogenic diet and that includes cutting back on the sweet stuff, sugar. So, if you can't use sugar to sweeten the deal, what can you use? Low-carb sweeteners are about to become your heroes. We're going to give you a list of keto-friendly sweeteners you can use and some that you should steer clear of.

Erythritol

Erythritol is a natural type of alcohol sugar that tricks your taste buds into experiencing the taste of sugar. There are approximately 4g of carbs in a teaspoon and about 0.2 calories in a gram of erythritol. It has to be said that this sweetener is not as nearly as potent as other sweeteners, it is only around 80% the sweetness of regular sugar. You can use erythritol for both cooking and baking.

You can use erythritol instead of sugar at a ratio of 1:1.33 by replacing every 100g of normal sugar with 133g of erythritol. It's also worthwhile remembering that this sweetener doesn't completely dissolve like sugar and will give your food and drink a gritty feeling.

Monk Fruit Sweetener

Monk fruit is a plant from southern China and it is used to create a natural sweetener that takes its name from its origin, monk fruit sweetener. Contrary to how sweetness works in other fruits, it's the antioxidants in monk fruit that give it the sweet taste. These antioxidants are found in the natural sugars called mogrosides within the fruit.

Mogrosides are naturally occurring in monk fruit but they are also variable in amount. This makes the extract anywhere between as sweet as sugar or sweetener depending on the mogroside concentration. This is an ideal sweetener for anyone following the ketogenic diet because it contains no carbohydrates or sugar. It is a good replacement to use in any situation you would use normal sugar. However, because of the variation in mogroside concentration the substitution may be anywhere from a 1:1 ratio to using only half the amount of sweetener as you would regular sugar.

Important note: The amount of monk fruit sweetener you use will depend on the brand and what additional ingredients are added to the product. Sometimes monk fruit extract is mixed with other sweeteners or even sugar or molasses which will increase the carbohydrate and calorie content of the product.

Stevia

Stevia is as natural as they come since it comes from the Stevia rebaudiana plant. It's perfect for a keto diet as it is essentially non-nutritive, containing almost no carbohydrates or calories. You can pick it up from your local supermarket in both powdered and liquid forms and it may be used to add some sweetness to a variety of foods and drinks from coffee to baking.

Important note: You need to use less stevia to sweeten food or drink because it is much sweeter than regular sugar. For example, if a recipe calls for 200g of regular sugar, only use 4 grams of stevia powder.

Sucralose

Unlike stevia, sucralose is an artificial compound. Your body isn't able to metabolize sucralose so it just passes through without adding to your carb or calorie count. Sucralose, the ingredient, might be free of calories but that doesn't mean it isn't mixed in with other ingredients by the time it reaches your table or kitchen. Splenda is a well-known brand of sweetener with a sucralose base but it's also mixed with dextrose and maltodextrin. These ingredients are carbohydrates that do add calories and carbs to the final product.

Important note: Sucralose is not a good sugar substitute for baking due to the high temperatures; it should be used for sweetening food and drink that is not subjected to such high temperatures. Sucralose-based sweeteners, like Splenda, can be used to substitute sugar at a ratio of 1:1 by replacing sugar with an equal amount of sweetener. If you are using pure sucralose, you only need to use a small fraction of the amount of sugar you would normally use as pure sucralose is extremely potent.

Xylitol

Similar to erythritol, xylitol is a sugar alcohol and is often used in sugar-free gum. Unlike erythritol, this sweetener is as sweet as sugar and also has only one carb and three calories per gram. However, if one carb per gram sounds less than ideal, there's good news. Being sugar alcohol, the carbohydrates in xylitol don't raise insulin or blood sugar levels as much as regular sugar so they don't count as net carbs.

Xylitol can be used to sweeten a variety of food and drink items, including baked goodies. However, it tends to absorb moisture so extra liquid should be added when using xylitol in baking to prevent dryness. When substituting xylitol for sugar, use a 1:1 ratio by replacing the amount of sugar with the same amount of sweetener.

Important note: Xylitol may cause digestive problems, especially if ingested in higher quantities. It is important to pay attention to any negative reactions and cut back on how much you use if you experience any side effects.

Yacon Syrup

The yacon plant is a South American tuber and the syrup made from this plant is used as an alternative to sugar. The syrup is packed with a soluble fiber that the human body cannot digest, fructooligosaccharides (FOS), as well as a few simple sugars such as glucose, fructose, and sucrose. The high indigestible soluble fiber content of the syrup means that this sweetener contains only one-third of the caloric value of sugar.

Yacon syrup contains about 20 calories and 11 grams of carbohydrates per tablespoon. It can be substituted at a 1:1 ratio for other liquid sweeteners such as cane juice, corn syrup, or molasses.

Important note: Yacon syrup can be used to replace sugar in tea, coffee, etc. However, it is not recommended as a sweetener when cooking because the soluble fiber may break down when subjected to high heat.

Main Ingredients Used in This Book

There is a huge variety of keto ingredients available but for this book, the following ingredients were used for most of the recipes concentrating on freely available ingredients and easy to use for all bakers from beginnings to experienced bakers.

Flour

- Almond flour
- Coconut flour
- Psyllium husk powder

Cheeses

- Cream cheese
- Mozzarella
- Cheddar

Dairy

- Eggs
- Butter
- Sour cream
- Heavy cream

Oil

- Olive oil
- Vegetable oil of personal preference

Sugar Substitutes

- Erythritol
- Xylitol

Before going to the recipes, I would like to ask you to kindly review this book if you enjoyed it, or if you have constructive criticism, I am looking forward to receiving your review.

Enjoy your cooking!

CHAPTER 3: EASY BREAD MACHINE RECIPES

All the bread machine recipes are easy to make using the minimum of ingredients.

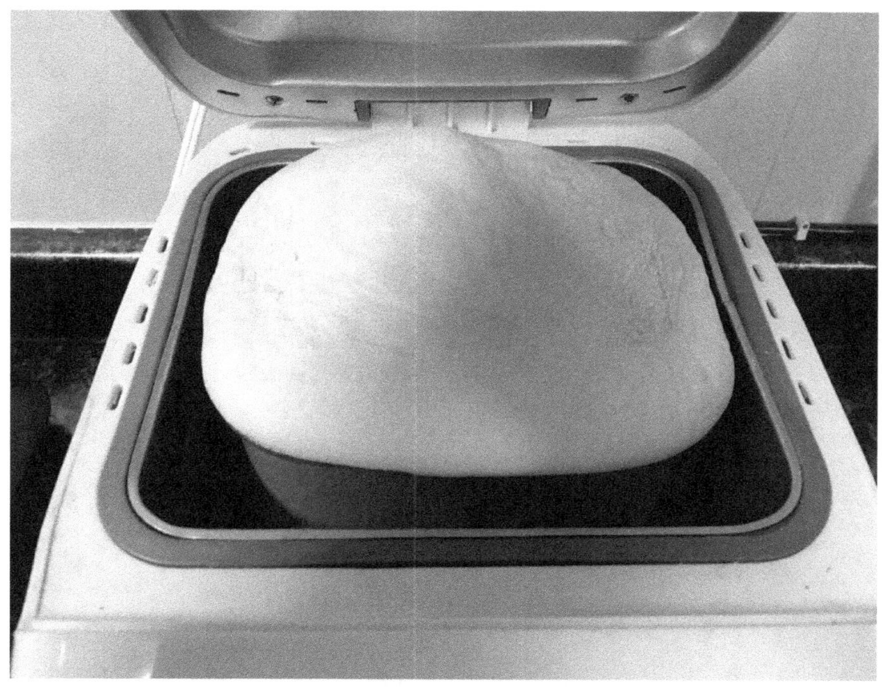

Low-Carb Carbalose Flour Bread

Prep Time: 10 minutes

Cook Time: basic or low-carb setting

Serving Size: 12 slices, 1 slice per serving

Nutritional Facts/Info per serving:

Calories 57 Kcal
Carbs 2 g
Fat 5 g
Protein 1 g

Ingredients

- 3 cups carbalose flour (any low-carb flour can be used, but nutritional value will differ)
- 3 tsp Vital wheat gluten
- 1 ½ tsp yeast for bread machines
- 1 ½ Tbsp sugar
- 1 cup warm water (not boiling)
- 1.4 cup vegetable oil of own choice

Instructions

1. Lightly spray the pan with vegetable oil of your own choice and set it aside.
2. Place the yeast, sugar, and warm water into the bread machine pan and leave for about 10 minutes to activate. It is ready when it forms bubbles.
3. Add the rest of the ingredients to the yeast mixture in the pan and bake using the basic setting or the low-card mode.
4. Once the bread is done, remove it from the pan and allow it to cool down slightly before slicing.

Notes

1. The sugar may be omitted, but it will change the texture and the taste of the bread.
2. You can use any low-carb flour of your own choice, but it will change the nutritional values.
3. To make the bread gluten-free, use gluten-free low-carb flour.

Oat Fiber and Flaxseed Meal Bread

Prep Time: 10 minutes

Cook Time: regular setting

Serving Size: 1 loaf, 16 slices, 1 slice per serving

Nutritional Facts/Info per serving:

Calories 155
Carbs 3 g net
Fat 5 g
Protein 13 g

Ingredients

- 1 ¼ cup Vital wheat gluten
- ½ cup oat fiber
- ⅔ cup flaxseed meal
- 1 Tbsp active dry yeast (Don't use any other type)
- ¼ cup Xylitol
- 1 tsp salt
- ½ tsp xanthan gum
- 2 eggs beaten well
- 1 Tbsp butter at room temperature
- 1 cup water at room temperature
- 1 tsp honey

Instructions

1. Lightly grease the inside of the bread machine bowl and set it aside.
2. Place the beaten egg, water. butter, and honey into the bread machine bowl.
3. Place all the dry ingredients, except the dry yeast, into a mixing bowl and whisk to combine.
4. Place the dry ingredients mixture on top of the wet mixture into the bread machine bowl.
5. Lastly, sprinkle the dry yeast over the ingredients in the bowl.
6. Close the bread machine and bake at the regular setting.
7. This is moist bread, so allow the bread to cool down before slicing.

Notes

1. The honey is needed to feed and activate the yeast and should not be left out.
2. Only trace amounts of the honey are present in the baked loaf and this has been calculated into the carbohydrate count.
3. This bread is well suited to toasting.

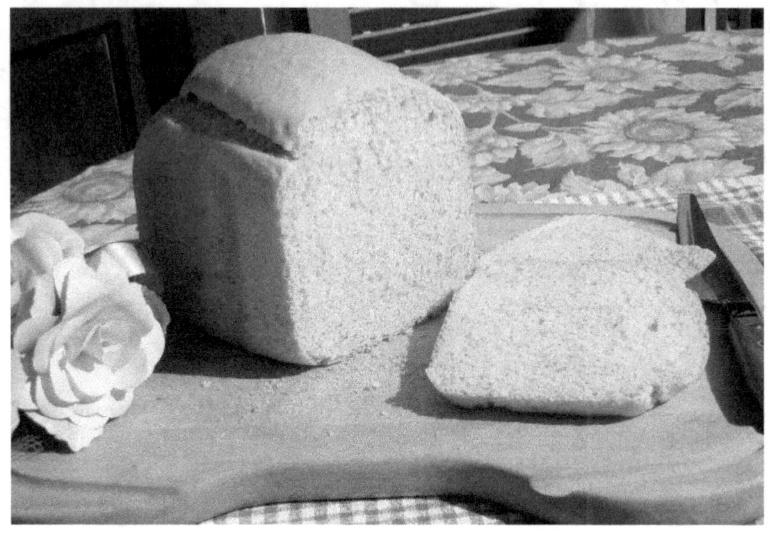

Yeast Bread

Prep Time: 5 minutes

Cook Time: 4 hours

Serving Size: 1 loaf, 16 slices, 1 slice per serving

Nutritional Facts/Info per serving:

Calories 99 Kcal
Carbs 7 g
Fat 5 g
Protein 9 g

Ingredients

- ¼ cup oat flour
- ¼ cup flax meal
- 1 cup Vital wheat gluten flour
- ¾ cup soy flour
- 1 cup wheat brand, coarse and unprocessed
- 1 package rapid rise/highly active dry yeast
- 1 ⅛ cup water, warm (120 - 130 F)
- ½ tsp sugar (see notes)

- 1 Tbsp sugar Splenda or sugar substitute of own choice
- 3 Tbsp olive oil
- 1 tsp salt
- 1 ½ tsp baking powder

Instructions

1. Place the yeast, water, and sugar in the bottom of the bread machine pan and stir. Proof the yeast until it forms bubbles.
2. Put the vital wheat gluten flour, flax meal, oil, soy flour, oat flour, wheat bran, baking powder, sweetener, and salt into a medium-sized mixing bowl and combine.
3. Pour the mixture over the yeast mixture in the bread machine pan.
4. Bake the bread on the basic cycle of the bread machine (3 - 4 hours).
5. Place the bread on a cooling rack to cool down and slice into 16 even slices.

Notes

1. It is not essential to proof the dry yeast, but this process confirms whether the yeast is active or not as inactive yeast will not bubble. You can skip the proofing by putting the yeast, water, and sugar into the bread pan and immediately add the rest of the ingredients as per the instructions above.
2. The sugar is not counted for the nutrition values as it is consumed by the yeast.
3. Almond flour can be substituted for soy flour without affecting the taste or texture of the bread.

Almond Flour Quick Bread (Gluten-Free, Paleo)

Prep Time: 10 minutes

Cook Time: 1 hour

Serving Size: 1 loaf, 18 slices, 1 ½ inch thick slice

Nutritional Facts/Info per serving:

Calories 123 Kcal
Carbs 5 g
Fat 10 g
Protein 4 g

Ingredients
- ¼ cup psyllium husk powder
- 2 cups almond flour (blanched)
- ½ salt
- 1 Tbsp gluten-free baking powder
- ¼ cup coconut oil (measure before melting)
- 4 eggs large, beaten
- ½ cup water warm

Instructions

1. Place all the ingredients into the bread machine bowl.
2. For the best results follow your bread machine manufacturer manual and place the ingredients into the bowl in the order advised in the manual.
3. If your bread machine manual does not provide instructions, the rule to follow is to place the wet ingredients in first, followed by the dry ingredient, and add the baking powder in last.
4. Bake the bread at the quick bread setting.
5. Place bread on a cooling rack and then slice the loaf into 18 equal slices.

Notes

1. Psyllium husk powder can turn the bread purple, but it does not affect the taste.

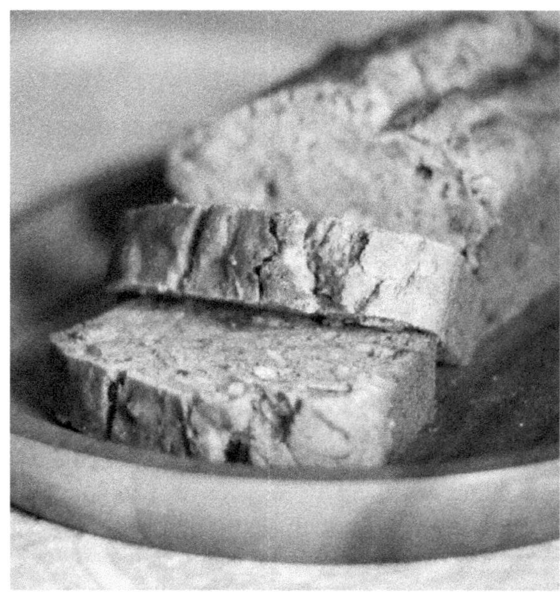

Wheat Gluten Flour and Soy Bread

Prep Time: 5 minutes

Cook Time: 2 hours

Serving Size: 1 loaf makes 11 slices and 1 slice per serving

Nutritional Facts/Info per serving:

Calories 76
Carbs 3.5 g
Fat 3.5 g
Protein 8.2 g

Ingredients
- 1 cup flax seeds ground
- ¾ cup Vital wheat gluten flour
- 1 cup soy flour
- 1 Tbsp Splenda sweetener
- 1 egg beaten
- ½ cup water
- 1 tsp dry yeast
- 1 Tbsp butter or margarine

Instructions

1. Combine all the ingredients in the bowl of the bread machine according to the instructions given in your bread machine manual.
2. Bake the bread on the light brown setting.
3. Allow the loaf to cool down in the bowl before removing it.
4. Slice into 11 slices and serve.

Notes

1. The sliced bread can be stored in the refrigerator in an airtight container.
2. During the last 15 minutes of the baking cycle, the lid of the bread machine might lift slightly. This is normal and once the bread is fully baked, the lid will lower again.
3. This bread toasts very well.

CHAPTER 4: GLUTEN-FREE BREAD

Gluten-free bread recipes are important to accommodate people with gluten intolerance and each of the recipes in this chapter address those needs. We have included gluten-free recipes in the other chapters as well for a bigger variety of gluten-free bread recipes.

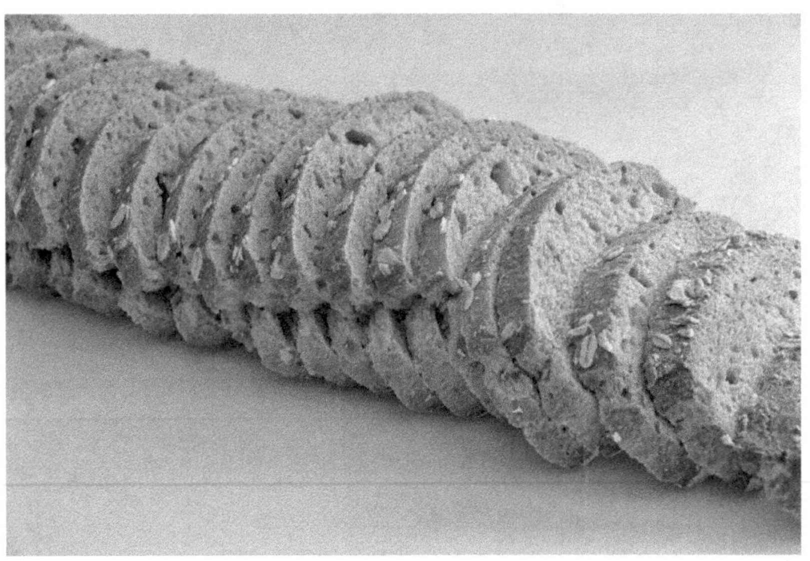

Almond Flour Yeast Bread

Prep Time: 10 minutes

Cook Time: 30 minutes

Serving Size: 1 loaf, makes 16 slices, 1 slice per serving

Nutritional Facts/Info per serving:

Calories 140 Kcal
Carbs 3 g
Fat 13 g
Protein 3 g

Ingredients

- 2 ⅛ cup almond flour
- 1 Tbsp psyllium husk powder
- ½ cup butter, unsalted and melted
- 1 tsp Inulin
- 1 tsp baking powder
- 2 tsp dry yeast
- 2 Tbsp water, warm
- 1 pinch salt
- 7 eggs, large
- ½ tsp xanthan gum

Instructions

1. Preheat the oven to 340 F (170 C).
2. Prepare a 9 x 5in loaf pan by spraying the pan with vegetable oil of your own choice and lining it with parchment paper. Set aside.
3. Place the inulin and yeast into a small mixing bowl.
4. Add the warm water to the mixing bowl and mix well.
5. Sit yeast mixture aside for 10 minutes in a warm place for the yeast to prove.
6. Place the psyllium, almond flour, xanthan gum, baking powder, and salt into a large mixing bowl and mix well.
7. Add the eggs and melted butter to the dry ingredients and mix until combined well.
8. Add the proofed yeast to the large mixing bowl and mix to combine.
9. Pour the mixture into the prepared loaf pan and cover with a tea towel.
10. Allow the batter to prove in a warm spot for 20 minutes.
11. Bake in the preheated oven for 30-40 minutes.
12. The bread is done when you hear a hollow sound when you tap the bread with your fingers and the crust is golden brown.
13. Remove the bread from the baking pan and place it on a cooling rack to cool down before slicing.

Notes

1. Store the bread in an airtight container in the refrigerator to use later.
2. The sliced bread can be stored in the freezer in resealable plastic bags for up to 3 months.

Soft-Textured Seed Bread

Prep Time: 10 minutes

Cook Time: 45 minutes

Serving Size: 1 loaf, makes 20 slices, 1 slice per serving

Nutritional Facts/Info per serving:

Calories Kcal 215
Carbs 2 g
Fat 19 g
Protein 6 g

Ingredients

- ¾ cup coconut flour
- 1 cup almond flour
- ¼ cup psyllium husk powder
- ½ cup flaxseed
- ⅓ cup sesame seeds
- 6 eggs
- 1 ⅓ cups cream cheese brought to room temperature
- ¾ cup of whipping cream heavy
- ½ cup of butter or coconut oil melted
- 3 tsp baking powder
- 1 tsp salt
- 1 tsp fennel or caraway seeds ground
- 1 Tbsp poppy or sesame seeds to use as a topping

Instructions

1. Preheat the oven to 350 F (180 C).
2. Prepare a loaf pan of about 4 x 7 inches and spray with vegetable oil (this may be omitted). Then line the bread pan with parchment paper.
3. Place all the dry ingredients into a mixing bowl, except the seeds that you will use for the topping.
4. Place the rest of the ingredients into a separate mixing bowl and whisk until the mixture has a smooth consistency.
5. Add the wet mixture to the bowl holding the dry ingredients and mix thoroughly.
6. Place the dough into the prepared loaf pan and then sprinkle the seeds on top.
7. Place on the lower rack in the oven and back for 45 minutes.
8. Test the bread with a skewer or knife. The bread is done if the skewer comes out clean.
9. Remove the bread from the baking pan. Do not let the bread cool down in the pan as this will cause the crust to become soggy.
10. Place the bread on a cooling rack and remove the parchment paper.
11. Allow the bread to cool down completely before slicing as this is moist bread and will crumble if sliced when hot.
12. Serve with toppings of your own choice.

Notes

1. The parchment paper can be omitted if you use non-stick baking pans.
2. This bread is suitable for sandwiches and toast.
3. You can store this bread for up to 5 days in the refrigerator in an airtight container.
4. It is suitable for freezing. For the best results, slice the bread before freezing and either freeze slices in individual bags or place parchment paper between the slices as this makes using single servings much easier. Frozen bread can be thawed in the refrigerator or at room temperature.

Nut-Free Coconut Flour Bread

Prep Time: 10 minutes

Cook Time: 50 minutes

Serving Size: 1 loaf, makes 16 slices, 1 slice per serving

Nutritional Facts/Info per serving:

Calories 95 Kcal
Carbs 2 g
Fat 9 g
Protein 3 g

Ingredients

- ½ cup Coconut flour
- 7 eggs, large
- ½ tsp xanthan gum
- ½ cup butter (to make bread dairy-free use ½ cup coconut or olive oil)
- ¼ tsp baking powder
- ¼ tsp salt

Instructions

1. Preheat oven to 355 F (180 C)
2. Line an 8.5 x 5 inches loaf pan with parchment paper.
3. Crack the eggs into a mixing bowl and mix until well combined, about 1 minute.
4. Add the butter, xanthan gum, coconut flour, baking powder, and salt to the egg mixture and mix until all the ingredients are combined. The mixture is quite thick, this is normal.
5. Pour the bread batter into the prepared loaf pan and smooth the top with a spatula.
6. Place on the middle rack in the oven and bake for 50 minutes.
7. Test to see if the bread is done by inserting a skewer into the middle of the bread. It is done when the skewer comes out clean.
8. Turn loaf out onto a cooling rack and allow the bread to cool down slightly before slicing.

Notes

1. Please note that regular baking powder can react with coconut flour and cause a greenish tint to the bread. To prevent this, shop for aluminum-free baking powder.
2. To make the bread dairy-free, substitute the butter with olive oil or any vegetable oil of your own choice.
3. The bread can be stored safely for up to 5 days in the fridge and can be frozen for up to 2 weeks, seal the bread in individual portions before freezing.

Sandwich Bread (Paleo and Keto)

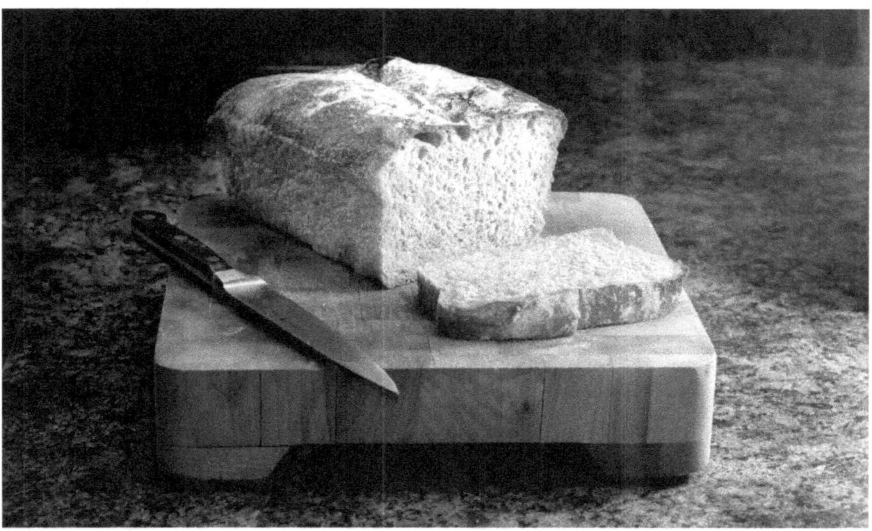

Prep Time: 8 minutes

Cook Time: 75 minutes

Serving Size: 1 loaf, makes 24 slices, 1 slice per serving

Nutritional Facts/Info per serving:
Calories 297 Kcal
Carbs 22 g
Fat 21 g
Protein 8 g

Ingredients

- 1 ½ cups tapioca flour
- 2 cups almond flour
- 2 Tbsp psyllium husk powder
- 1 cup golden flax meal, milled
- 8 eggs, large
- ¾ cup melted coconut oil
- ½ cup water
- 1 tsp salt
- 4 tsp baking powder
- 1 Tbsp apple cider vinegar

Instructions

1. Preheat the oven to 350 F (180 C).
2. Prepare a 4 x 8 inches bread pan by greasing it, or lining the bread pan with parchment paper.
3. You can use a high-speed electric mixer, a food processor, or hand mix the ingredients for this bread.
4. Combine all the ingredients and mix until you have smooth bread dough.
5. Scrape the dough into the prepared bread pan and place it into the oven on the middle rack.
6. Bake for 1 hour 15 minutes and test the bread with a skewer to see if it is done. When the skewer comes out clean the bread is ready and can be removed from the oven.
7. Place the bread on a cooling rack to cool down, then slice into 24 equal-sized slices.

Notes

4. This loaf can be stored in the refrigerator for 3 days in a sealable container.
5. Suitable for freezing and after defrosting can be used as it or toasted.

Low-Carb Mini Cheese Loaves (Gluten-Free, Paleo, Keto)

Prep Time: 38 minutes (includes chill time)

Cook Time: 10 - 12 minutes

Serving Size: 4 servings, 2 mini loaves per serving

Nutritional Facts/Info per serving:

Calories Kcal 281
Carbs 6 g
Fat 22 g
Protein 15 g

Ingredients

- ¼ cup cream cheese
- ¾ cup mozzarella cheese, shredded
- ⅓ cup almond flour or coconut flour
- ⅓ tsp garlic powder
- 2 tsp baking powder
- 1 beaten egg
- ½ tsp Italian seasoning
- ½ cup cheddar cheese, shredded

Instructions

1. Preheat the oven to 425 F (220 C).
2. Grease a flat baking pan and set it aside.
3. Place the cream cheese and mozzarella cheese in a microwave-safe bowl and microwave on high for 1 minute. Stir the mixture every 20 seconds until completely melted.
4. Place the baking powder, almond fl9our, Italian seasoning, garlic powder, and egg into a mixing bowl and combine.
5. Stir the melted cheese mixture into the dry ingredients until fully combined.
6. Lastly, stir in the cheddar cheese and shape the dough into a ball.
7. Cover the dough ball and chill in the refrigerator for 30 minutes.

8. Use almond flour to dust a cutting board and cut the dough ball into 4 equal-sized pieces and roll each piece into a ball.
9. Cut each of the 4 balls into two even-sized pieces and place them on the greased baking pan with the cut side placed down on the baking pan.
10. Bake for 10 - 12 minutes. The mini loaves are done when they are golden brown.
11. Serve warm or cold with fillings of your own choice.

Notes

1. Instead of 8 mini loaves (2 per serving), make 2 balls cut into half. This gives you 4 larger mini loaves with 1 loaf per serving.
2. This cheese bread dough is suitable to be used for pizza crusts as well. The baking time for the crusts is about the same as for the mini loaves and can be topped with ingredients of your own choice. Place the crusts back into the oven after adding the toppings and bake for about 7 minutes.

CHAPTER 5: CHEESE BREAD

Cheese in its many forms plays a large role in keto diets and these recipes all use popular and easily available cheese types.

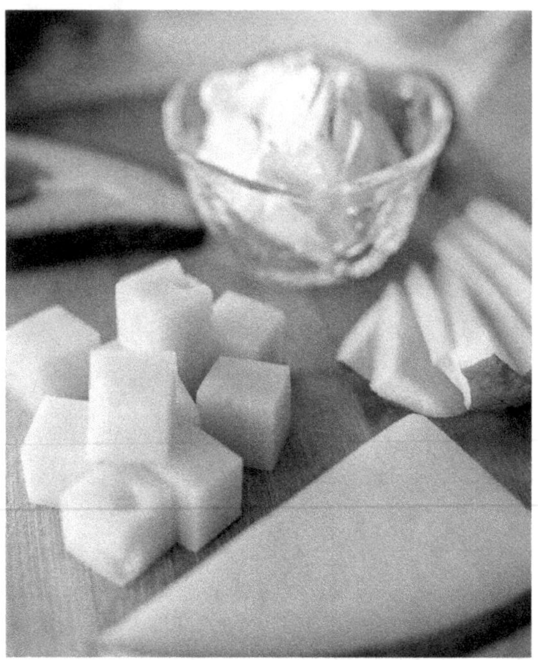

Cream Cheese Bread

Prep Time: 10 minutes

Cook Time: 40 minutes

Serving Size: 1 loaf, 12 slices, 1 slice per serving

Nutritional Facts/Info per serving:

Calories 102 Kcal
Carbs 1.9 g
Fat 9.6 g
Protein 3.1 g

Ingredients

- ½ cup cream cheese, full fat (important to see notes below about the cream cheese)
- 1 ¼ cup almond flour, finely milled
- 2 tsp baking powder
- 1 Tbsp sugar substitute, optional (see notes)
- 4 eggs
- 3 Tbsp butter, unsalted, and at room temperature
- ½ salt

Instructions

1. Preheat the oven to 350 F (180 C).
2. Grease an 8 inches bread pan and set it aside.
3. Measure and sift the almond flour into a medium-sized mixing bowl and add the baking powder and salt and set the bowl aside.
4. Place the butter and the sugar substituted into a large mixing bowl. Use an electric mixer at high speed to blend until the mixture is fluffy and light.
5. Add the eggs to the butter mixture one at a time and mix well after each egg is added using the electric mixer on medium-low.
6. Then add the dry ingredients from the medium mixing bowl into the butter and egg mixture using the low setting on an electric mixer. Make sure that the batter is fully combined.
7. Pour the batter into the prepared loaf pan and bake until the top of the loaf is golden brown, about 30 - 40 minutes.
8. Test the bread by inserting a toothpick into the bread. The bread is done when the toothpick comes out clean.
9. Leave the loaf in the baking pan to cool down for 10 minutes, then turn the loaf out onto a cooling rack to cool down completely before slicing.

Notes

1. It is important to use the full-fat cream cheese that comes in a brick. Using the whipped low-fat cream cheese available in tubs will change the outcome of the bread drastically and most likely the bread will be a flop.
2. Using sugar substitute is optional, but it gives the bread the flavor of and taste of conventional white bread.
3. This bread can be made into cheese rolls. Place even quantities into a 12-cup muffin pan and bake for 20 - 25 minutes. Makes 12 rolls and 1 roll is a serving.
4. This cream cheese bread can be stored for up to 7 days in the fridge either as a whole loaf, or sliced in an airtight container.
5. This bread is suitable to be frozen as slices or as a whole loaf for up to 30 days. Make sure that you cover the bread well before putting it in the freezer.

Cheese, Bacon and Garlic Bread

One of my favorites.

Prep Time: 15 minutes

Cook Time: 20 minutes

Serving Size: 6 servings, 1 bread ball per serving

Nutritional Facts/Info per serving:

Calories 127 Kcal
Carbs 1.98 g
Fat 9.7 g
Protein 8.5 g

Ingredients

- ¼ cup cream cheese
- 2 ½ cups shredded mozzarella cheese
- ½ cup parmesan cheese, grated
- 3 eggs

- 1 ½ cups super-fine almond flour
- ⅓ cup bacon bits, cooked
- 1 tsp Italian seasoning
- 1 tsp baking powder

Garlic Sauce

- 4 finely minced garlic cloves
- ¼ butter, browned (see notes)
- ½ cup fresh chopped parsley

Instructions

1. Preheat the oven to 400 F (200 C).
2. Prepare a medium cast-iron skillet by spraying the inside with vegetable oil (see notes).
3. Put the Italian seasoning and parmesan cheese in a shallow dish or a plate and combine.
4. Melt the cream cheese and mozzarella cheese in a microwave-proof bowl for 1 minute in the microwave on high and mix well with a spatula.
5. Add the eggs, almond flour, baking powder, and bacon bits to the melted cheese and combine until the mixture is smooth.
6. Make 6 evenly-sized dough balls using a large cookie scoop or large serving spoon and place each ball into the Italian seasoning and parmesan cheese mixture to coat all around.
7. Place the bread balls into the cast iron skillet and sprinkle any leftover seasoning over the top and add extra parmesan cheese (optional).
8. Place the skillet with the bread balls in the refrigerator to chill for 10 minutes.
9. Place the skillet onto the center rack in the oven and bake until bread is golden brown, 20 to 25 minutes.
10. Remove skillet from the oven and liberally brush the garlic butter sauce over the bread and serve warm or cold.

Notes

1. Brown the butter for the garlic sauce by placing it into a saucepan and melting the butter. Keep it on the heat until the butter turns a very light brown. Browning the butter creates a nutty flavor that is missing when melting butter normally.
2. If you don't have a cast-iron skillet, you can use a round oven-proof glass dish.

Cheddar Cheese Loaf

Prep Time: 10 minutes

Cook Time: 30 minutes

Serving Size: 1 loaf, makes 12 slices, 1 slice per serving

Nutritional Facts/Info per serving:

Calories 120 Kcal
Carbs 5.3 g
Fat 7.8 g
Protein 9 g

Ingredients
- 2 cups almond flour
- 2 tsp baking powder
- 1 ½ cups whey protein isolate that does not contain additives
- 2 tsp xanthan gum
- 1 tsp oregano
- ½ tsp salt (or to taste)
- 1 ½ Tbsp onion powder
- 2 Tbsp garlic powder
- ½ tsp chili flakes (this is optional)
- 1 tsp dried parsley
- 1 cup warm water (max 110 F)
- 1 cup cheddar cheese, shredded

Instructions

1. Preheat the oven to 375 F (190 C).
2. Line an 8 x 4 inches bread pan with parchment paper or use a silicone pan sprayed with vegetable oil.
3. Place the almond flour, salt, protein powder, xanthan gum, baking powder, garlic powder, oregano, parsley, onion powder, and chili flakes into a large mixing bowl and whisk together.
4. Add the warm water to the mixing bowl and mix thoroughly with a spatula.
5. Lastly, add the cheddar cheese and stir to combine.
6. Pour the bread batter into the prepared loaf pan.
7. Bake on the middle rack of the oven for 30 minutes.
8. Place the loaf on a cooling rack and slice it into 12 slices once the bread has cooled down.

Notes

1. Optional herbs and spices can be added as per personal preference.
2. The bread is suitable for toasting and can be stored in the fridge for 3 days, or frozen for up to 30 days in portions in foil, or wrapped in wax paper, or placed in sealable plastic bags.

Sharp Cheddar Cheese Beer Bread (Gluten-Free)

Prep Time: 5 minutes

Cook Time: 55 minutes

Serving Size: 1 loaf, 12 slices, 1 slice per serving

Nutritional Facts/Info per serving:

Calories 222 Kcal
Carbs 6 g
Fat 19 g
Protein 9 g

Ingredients

- 2 cups almond flour, super fine
- 1 ½ Tbsp oat fiber
- 3 Tbsp granulated sweetener
- 1 Tbsp baking powder
- 4 beaten eggs, large
- ½ cup light beer
- ¼ cup olive oil, extra virgin
- ½ tsp salt
- 1 ¼ cup sharp cheddar cheese, shredded (divided)

Instructions

1. Preheat the oven to 350 F (180 C).
2. Liberally grease a standard loaf pan (4 x 8 inches).
3. Sift all the dry ingredients into a large mixing bowl.
4. Add all the wet ingredients to the bowl and stir with a spoon or a spatula until the mixture is smooth.
5. Add 1 cup of cheddar cheese to the mixture and fold in.
6. Scrape the bread batter into the prepared loaf pan and use a spatula to smooth the top.

7. Sprinkle the last ¼ cup of cheddar cheese over the top.
8. Place the bread pan on the middle rack in the oven and bake for 45 - 55 minutes.
9. Cover the bread pan with aluminum foil after 30 minutes. Make a tent over the bread pan, do not press the foil down onto the bread. This is to prevent the bread from browning too fast or too much.
10. Test the bread by inserting a toothpick into the middle. It is done when the toothpick comes out clean.
11. Allow the loaf to cool down for 20 minutes in the pan.
12. Then place a large plate or a cutting board on top of the bread and invert the plate/ cutting board together with the loaf pan. This makes it easier for the loaf to be released from the pan.
13. Place the loaf on a cooling rack and only slice the bread into 12 slices once the bread has completely cooled down.

Notes

1. If you do not have oat fiber, add 1 ½ Tbsp of almond or coconut flour. The oat fiber is normally added as it improves the texture of the bread, but the substitutes work well.
2. The bread can be stored in the refrigerator for 4 - 5 days.

Bacon and Cheese Loaf

Prep Time: 12 minutes

Cook Time: 45 minutes

Serving Size: 1 loaf, 10 slices, 1 slice per serving

Nutritional Facts/Info per serving:

Calories 292 Kcal
Carbs 4 g
Fat 26 g
Protein 10 g

Ingredients

- 1 ½ cups almond flour
- 1 cup (8 oz) bacon, cooked (see notes for substitute ideas)
- 4 Tbsp melted butter, cooled down
- 1 cup cheddar cheese, mild or sharp
- 1 Tbsp baking powder
- 2 eggs
- ⅓ cup sour cream

Instructions

1. Preheat the oven to 300 F (150 C).
2. Grease and line a standard loaf pan (4 x 8 inches).
3. Cook the diced bacon in a frying pan until crisp (do not overcook the bacon).
4. Place the almond flour and baking powder into a medium-sized mixing bowl and whisk to break up any lumps in the almond flour.
5. Place the eggs and sour cream in a separate mixing bowl and whisk until smooth.
6. Combine the almond flour and cooked baking with the egg and cream mixture.
7. Add the melted butter to the mixture and fold in gently.

8. Pour the bread batter into the prepared bread pan and bake for 45 - 50 minutes. Test for readiness with a skewer and bread is done when the skewer comes out clean.

9. Important: do not slice the bread while it is still warm as it will crumble.

10. Place the cooled bread loaf in the fridge to cool down completely and then slice the loaf into 10 slices.

Notes

1. There are several substitutes for the bacon in this recipe that works well. Remember though, that it will affect your nutritional values and make allowances for that.

2. Prosciutto.

3. Ham.

4. Beef bacon.

5. Turkey bacon.

6. Pepperoni.

7. Smoked Italian sausage.

8. Smoked chicken strips.

9. For spicy bread, loaf add 1 - 2 chopped or sliced jalapenos or 1 - 2 tsp of chili flakes.

10. Optional toppings can be added such as extra shredded cheese or a sprinkling of your favorite herbs or spice mix before putting the loaf into the oven.

CHAPTER 6: SAVORY VEGETABLE LOAVES

Vegetables play an important part in keto diets and this chapter uses a variety of vegetables to cater to the tastes of everyone who loves vegetable loaves.

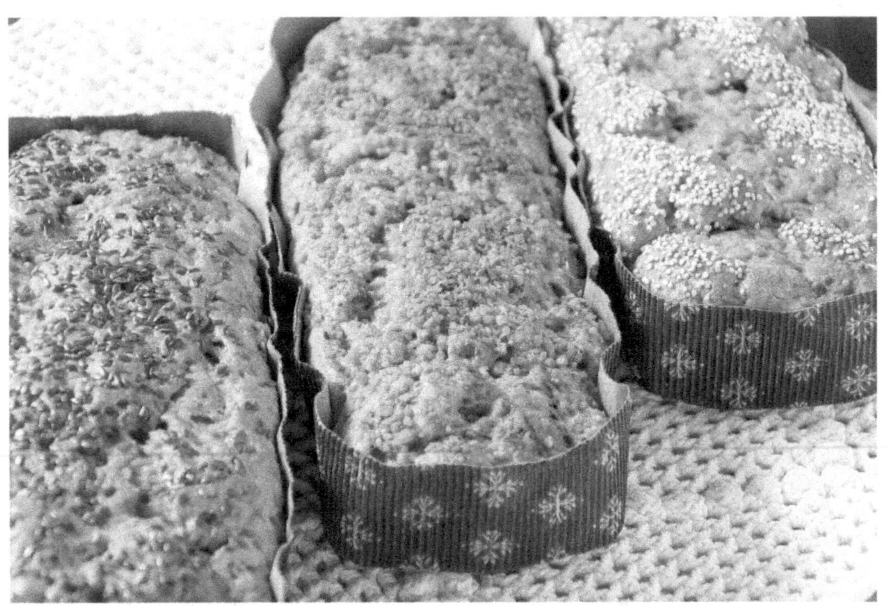

Gluten-Free Zucchini Bread or Muffins

Prep Time: 10 minutes

Cook Time: 1 hour

Serving Size: 1 loaf makes 12 slices, 1 slice per serving

Nutritional Facts/Info per serving:

Calories 166 Kcal
Carbs 5 g
Fat 15 g
Protein 6 g

Ingredients

- 2 cups almond flour
- 1 ½ cups zucchini, grated with the peel
- ½ tsp salt
- 1 tsp baking soda
- ¼ cup butter, melted
- 2 beaten eggs, large
- ½ cup granular sweetener (omit for savory bread, see notes)
- ½ tsp cinnamon, ground (omit for savory bread or muffins, see notes)

Instructions

1. Preheat the oven to 350 F (180 C).
2. Prepare a 0 x 5 inches loaf pan or 12 cup muffin pan by greasing with butter or spraying with vegetable oil.
3. Place the flour, baking soda, salt, sweetener, and cinnamon (for sweet option) in a mixing bowl and combine.
4. Place the grated zucchini on a cotton kitchen cloth and wrap it tightly. Then squeeze out and discard as much liquid as possible. Then add the dry zucchini to the dry ingredients.
5. Next, add the melted butter and eggs to the mixing bowl and stir until the batter is thoroughly combined. (See notes for optional extras to add to the batter).
6. Scrape the batter into the prepared loaf pan or scoop evenly into the muffin pan. Bake the loaf for 60 minutes. Bread is done when a skewer comes out clean.
7. If making muffins, then bake the muffins for 18 - 20 minutes and test with a toothpick to see if it is done.

Notes

1. This recipe can be made as savory bread or muffins or as sweet bread or muffins. When baking savory, omit the cinnamon and sweetener.
2. Optional ingredients such as blueberries (1 cup), walnuts (½ cup),

and chocolate chips (½ cup) can be added to the batter and add extra sweetness. Fold any optional ingredients into the batter just before baking. You must adjust the nutritional values if using optional extras.

3. This bread is suitable for freezing. Bread must be completely cooled down before freezing either as a loaf or individual slices. Wrap loaf or slices in plastic and then in foil and place in the freezer. Bread can be frozen for 4 months. For eating, defrost by putting bread on a kitchen counter, it defrosts quite fast.

Veggie Loaf (Gluten and Dairy Free)

Prep Time: 15 minutes

Cook Time: 55 - 70 minutes

Serving Size: 1 loaf makes 12 slices, 1 slice per serving

Nutritional Facts/Info per serving:

Calories 175 Kcal
Carbs 3.8 g
Fat 14.6 g
Protein 6.7 g

Ingredients

- ⅓ cup coconut flour
- 1 cup almond flour
- 2 Tbsp psyllium husks
- ½ cup seeds, mixed (pumpkin, sunflower, flax, and sesame seeds)
- 1 cup pumpkin, grated
- 2 ¼ cups (11 oz) grated zucchini
- ½ cup grated carrots
- ¼ cup of coconut oil or ghee
- 5 medium eggs or 4 extra-large eggs
- 2 tsp cumin, ground
- 1 Tbsp paprika, smoked
- 2 tsp salt, or as per personal preference
- 2 tsp baking powder
- 2 Tbsp mixed seeds extra, for garnish

Instructions

1. Preheat the oven to 340 F (170 C).
2. Prepare a standard-sized loaf pan by greasing it with butter or spraying it with vegetable oil.
3. Place the almond flour, salt, spices, coconut flour, baking powder, psyllium husks, and ½ cup of mixed seeds into a mixing bowl and combine.
4. Grate all the vegetables and put them onto a dry kitchen towel and wrap tightly. Wring the kitchen towel to extract as much moisture from the vegetables as possible.
5. Place the grated vegetables in a separate large mixing bowl and add the eggs and coconut oil/ghee and stir.
6. Add the dry ingredients to the veggie mixture and stir to combine. The mixture will look quite dry, this is normal.
7. Pour the bread mixture into the loaf pan and press the mixture down lightly. Lastly, sprinkle the 2 Tbsp mixed seeds on top of the bread batter.
8. Bake the bread uncovered on the middle rack in the oven until a skewer comes out clean, for 55 - 70 minutes.
9. Leave the loaf in the bread pan to cool down for 30 minutes and then place on a cooling rack to cool down completely.
10. Slice loaf into 12 slices and serve.

Notes

1. The ½ cup of mixed seeds can be replaced by mixed nuts of your choice.
2. Bread can be stored for up to 5 cays in the fridge. Reheat or toast the bread before serving.
3. Bread can be stored for up to 3 months in the freezer. Slice and individually wrap servings before freezing.

Olive Loaf (Gluten, Dairy, Soy Free, and Vegetarian)

Prep Time: 10 minutes

Cook Time: 45 minutes

Serving Size: 1 load, 10 slices, 1 slice per serving

Nutritional Facts/Info per serving:

Calories 240 Kcal
Carbs 8 g
Fat 19 g
Protein 11 g

Ingredients

- 6 eggs, large
- 3 Tbsp tapioca flour
- 2 ½ cups almond meal
- ¾ cup carbonated water
- 2 Tbsp dried herbs of own preference (oregano, rosemary, thyme)
- 2 tsp baking powder, gluten-free
- 12 large pitted olives, chopped
- 4 crushed garlic cloves
- pinch of salt

Instructions

1. Preheat the oven to 400 F (200 C).
2. Line a 4 x 8 inches loaf pan with parchment paper.
3. Whisk eggs in a large mixing bowl and add the carbonated water and whisk again.
4. Add the crushed garlic, olives, and herbs to the egg mixture and mix.
5. Add the tapioca flour, almond meal, salt, and baking powder and

mix until fully combined.

6. Pour the batter into the prepared loaf pan.
7. Place the bread pan on the center oven rack and bake for 45 minutes. Test with a toothpick to see if it is baked through.
8. Place the loaf on a cooling rack to cool down before serving.

Notes

1. The bread is suitable for sandwiches, as a dipping bread, and toasted.
2. The loaf can be stored in the fridge for up to 4 days.

Cauliflower Bread (Gluten-Free)

Prep Time: 10 minutes

Cook Time: 45 minutes

Serving Size: 1 loaf, 8 slices, 1 slice per serving

Nutritional Facts/Info per serving:

Calories 04 Kcal
Carbs 6 g
Fat 4 g
Protein 5 g

Ingredients

- 4 cups cauliflower rice (1 large head of cauliflower florets)
- 1 Tbsp psyllium husk powder
- 5 Tbsp coconut flour
- 4 eggs
- 2 Tbsp garlic powder
- 1 tsp salt
- 2 Tbsp onion powder
- ½ Tbsp baking powder

Instructions

1. Preheat the oven to 400 F (200 C).
2. Spray an 8 x 4 inches baking pan with vegetable oil and line the pan with parchment paper.
3. Blitz the cauliflower florets in a food processor only long enough to create cauliflower rice.
4. Place all the ingredients in a large mixing bowl and combine, but do not overmix the bread batter.
5. Scrape the bread batter into the prepared loaf pan using a spoon to press the batter down gently.
6. Bake for 45 minutes.
7. Place the bread on a cooling rack and allow it to cool down fully before slicing.

Notes

1. Bread can be stored in the fridge for up to 3 days and can be frozen for up to 30 days. Wrap each slice well before placing it in the freezer.
2. The psyllium husk powder can be substituted with ground chia seeds or ground flaxseed.

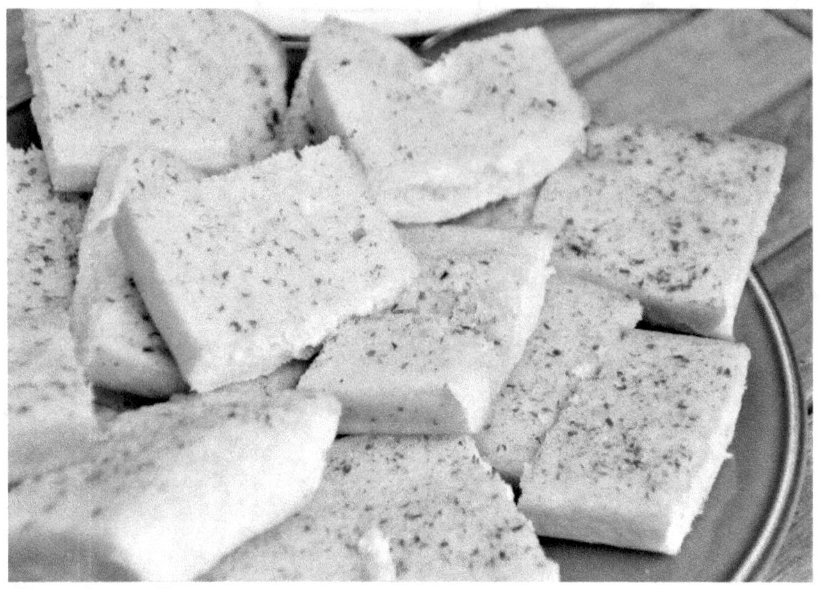

Cornbread

Prep Time: 10 minutes

Cook Time: 40 minutes

Serving Size: 1 loaf makes 12 slices, 1 slice per serving

Nutritional Facts/Info per serving:

Calories124 Kcal
Carbs 4 g
Fat 10 g
Protein 4 g

Ingredients

- ½ cup sifted coconut flour
- 1 can (15 oz) baby corn drained and puréed or chopped (see notes)
- 2 Tbsp sweetener powder, optional (see notes)
- 6 eggs
- ½ cup butter, unsalted (melt and cool down)
- ½ tsp salt
- 1 tsp baking powder

Instructions

1. Preheat the oven to 350 F (180 C).
2. Spray a 0 x 5 inches bread pan with vegetable oil or grease with butter.
3. Put the eggs and sweetener (if you are using this) into a mixing bowl and whisk to blend.
4. Pour the melted butter into the egg mixture while whisking.
5. Add the baby corn and stir.
6. Place the baking powder, coconut flour, and salt into a separate mixing bowl and stir to combine.
7. Add the flour mixture to the bowl holding the egg mixture and stir until the batter is fully combined.
8. Spoon the batter into the prepared bread pan.
9. Bake the cornbread for 40 minutes.
10. Allow the bread to cool down for 10 minutes or longer before slicing.
11. Spread butter on the slices and serve warm.
12. Let me know if you enjoyed it through a review :)

Notes

1. Fresh baby corn can be used instead of canned, using the same amount of fresh corn as there is in a 15-oz can.
2. If you prefer a cornbread that is not very sweet, you can omit the 2 Tbsp of sweetener powder.
3. The cornbread batter can also be used to make cornbread muffins. Use a 12 cup muffin pan and each muffin will be 1 serving. Baking time for muffins is 12 - 15 minutes and check with a toothpick to see if they are done.
4. For a spicy cornbread add cayenne powder, or chili flakes, or chopped chili peppers to personal preference.

CHAPTER 7: SWEET AND FRUIT LOAVES

When you follow the keto lifestyle, it does not mean you have to say goodbye to sweet bread loaves. You simply need recipes that are keto and delicious as snacks and dessert.

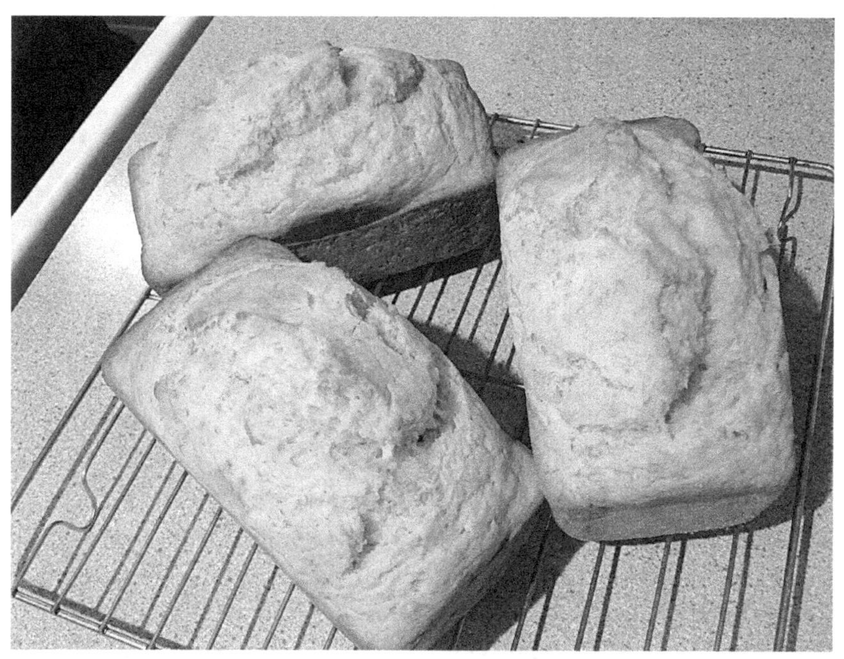

Banana Bread (Gluten and Grain Free)

Prep Time: 5 minutes

Cook Time: 40 minutes

Serving Size: 1 loaf makes 8 slices,1 slice per serving

Nutritional Facts/Info per serving:

Calories 205 Kcal
Carbs 6.4 g
Fat 17.2 g
Protein 8 g

Ingredients

- 1 ½ cup almond flour
- ¼ cup crushed walnuts (see notes for alternatives0
- ½ cup overripe banana, mashed
- 2 Tbsp melted butter
- 3 large eggs
- ¼ cup granulated erythritol (Swerve)
- 1 tsp baking powder
- 2 tsp cinnamon

Instructions

1. Preheat the oven to 356 F (180 C).
2. Line a 7 x 3.5 inches loaf pan with parchment paper and set it aside. (See notes).
3. Place the eggs, melted butter, and mashed banana into a mixing bowl and beat with an electric beater.
4. Place the almond flour, cinnamon, sweetener, and baking powder into a separate mixing bowl and stir to combine and then add dry mixture to the egg mixture and combine until the ingredients are fully blended.
5. Stir the crushed walnuts into the bread batter, keeping a small amount in reserve to sprinkle over the top of the bread.
6. Put the dough into the prepared baking pan and sprinkle the reserved walnuts evenly over the top.
7. Bake the loaf for 40 minutes until a test skewer comes out clean, but check the bread at 30 minutes, and if it is already brown, place aluminum over the bread pan loosely to prevent the bread from browning further or burning.
8. Allow the loaf to cool down completely before slicing.
9. Let me know if you enjoy it as much as I do :)

Notes

1. The walnuts can be replaced with any other nuts of your own choice and hazelnuts or pecans are recommended.
2. Sugar-free chocolate chips can be added as an optional extra.

3. A pinch of nutmeg can be added to the batter for extra flavor.
4. If you do not have a small loaf pan, you can double the recipe and use a 9 x 5 inches loaf pan. The baking time must then be increased to 55 - 60 minutes.
5. It is important to always use overripe bananas for this bread (the skin should have brown specks) as under-ripe or just ripe bananas have much less flavor.
6. To make this recipe dairy-free, use coconut oil instead of butter.

Moist Cinnamon Swirl Bread

Prep Time: 10 minutes

Cook Time: 1 hour

Serving Size: 1 loaf, 12 slices, 1 slice per serving

Nutritional Facts/Info per serving:

Calories 191 Kcal
Carbs 5 g
Fat 17 g
Protein 5 g

Ingredients

- 1 ½ cups almond flour
- ¼ cup coconut flour
- ½ cup sweetener (Swerve, Truvia, or Natvia)
- ½ melted butter, unsalted
- 1 tsp baking powder
- ½ cup almond milk, unsweetened
- 3 eggs, large
- 1 tsp vanilla essence
- ¼ cup sour cream
- 3 tsp ground cinnamon

Instructions

1. Preheat the oven to 350 F (180 C).
2. Grease or spray a 9 x 5 inches loaf pan with vegetable oil and then line the pan with parchment paper.
3. Put the coconut flour, almond flour, ⅓ cup of the sweetener, and baking powder into a large mixing bowl, and mix well.
4. Add the almond milk, butter, vanilla essence, eggs, and sour cream to the dry ingredients and mix to form a thick bread batter.
5. Put the remaining sweetener and cinnamon into a small bowl and mix.
6. Place half of the batter into the prepared loaf pan and sprinkle half of the cinnamon and sweetener mixture over the batter. Then spoon the rest of the batter into the loaf pan and top with the remaining cinnamon mixture.
7. Use a knife to create a swirl pattern through the batter.
8. Bake the bread on the middle rack in the oven for 55 - 65 minutes. The bread is done when it springs back when you press it with the back of a teaspoon.
9. Allow the bread to cool down in the bread pan for 10 minutes and then turn the loaf out onto a cooling rack to cool down completely.
10. Slice loaf into 12 slices and serve as is or add butter or topping of your own choice and serve.

Notes

1. The loaf can be stored in a covered container for up to 5 days in the fridge and can be frozen for up to 3 months.

Gluten-Free Ginger Loaf

Prep Time: 15 minutes

Cook Time: 25 - 30 minutes

Serving Size: 8 servings - 1 slice per serving

Nutritional Facts/Info per serving:

Calories 249 Kcal
Carbs 7.1 g
Fat 22.2 g
Protein 6.9 g

Ingredients for Loaf

- ¾ cup coconut flour
- 4 eggs, large
- 1 tsp baking powder, gluten-free
- ¼ cup unsalted butter, melted
- ¾ cup granulated erythritol or Swerve
- 2 Tbsp gingerbread spice mix (see below)
- 1 tsp vanilla extract, sugar-free

Ingredients for Icing

- ½ cup cream cheese softened
- 1 tsp vanilla extract, sugar-free
- ¼ cup powdered erythritol or Swerve
- ¼ cup walnuts, chopped (use toasted coconut flakes to make the loaf nut-free).

Ingredients for Gingerbread Spice Mix

- 2 tsp cinnamon, ground
- ½ tsp nutmeg, ground
- ¼ tsp salt
- 2 tsp ginger, ground
- ½ tsp allspice, ground
- ½ tsp cloves, ground

Instructions

1. Preheat the oven to 350 F (180 C) and for fan-assisted ovens to 310 F (155 C).
2. Grease with butter or spray an 8.5 x 4.6 x 2.5 inches loaf pan with vegetable oil and set aside.
3. Put the melted butter, eggs, and vanilla extract into a large mixing bowl and whisk.
4. Add the coconut flour, granulated sugar substitute, ginger spice mix, and baking powder to the egg mixture. Do not overmix the batter, just combine ingredients until they are mixed.
5. Put the batter into the prepared loaf pan and bake on the center rack in the oven for 25 - 30 minutes. If you use a narrower, regular loaf pan, adjust the baking time upward to 40 - 45 minutes.
6. The bread is done when it is golden brown and a test toothpick inserted into the loaf comes out clean.
7. Leave the bread in the baking pan until it has completely cooled down.
8. Place all the icing ingredients (except the walnuts) into a small bowl and use a hand beater to beat until all the ingredients are fully combined.
9. Spoon the icing onto the top of the loaf and even the icing out with a butter knife or spatula and sprinkle the walnuts on top of the icing.
10. Slice the gingerbread loaf into 7 even slices and serve.

Notes

1. The gingerbread can be stored in the refrigerator for 5 days in an airtight container.
2. The gingerbread can only be frozen without the icing. The plain gingerbread loaf can be frozen for up to 3 months.

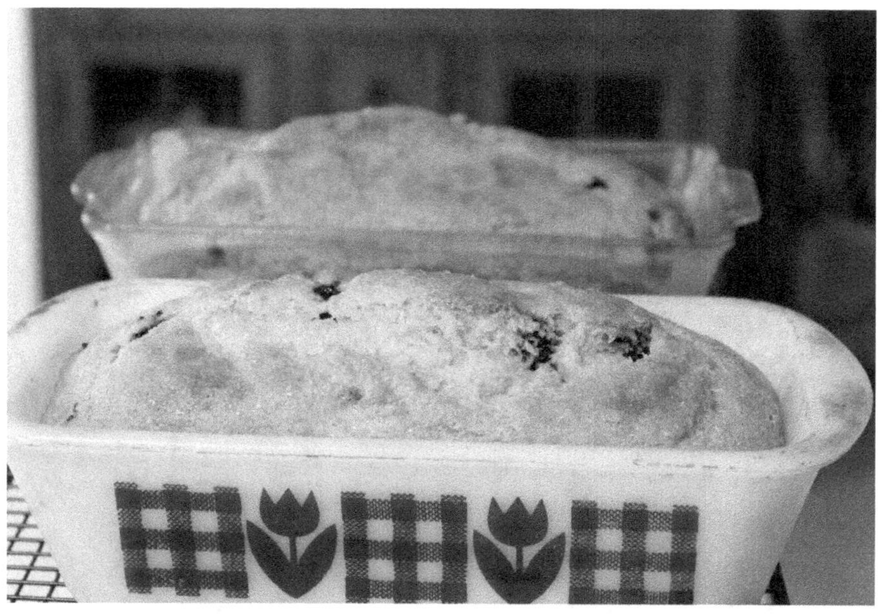

Blueberry and Lemon Bread (Dairy-Free)

Prep Time: 15 minutes

Cook Time: 1 hour

Serving Size: 1 loaf, 16 slices, 1 slice per serving

Nutritional Facts/Info per serving:

Calories 186 Kcal
Carbs 5.5 g
Fat 11.7 g
Protein 4.7 g

Ingredients

- 2 cups almond flour
- 1 ½ tsp baking powder
- ¼ cup coconut flour
- 5 eggs, large at room temperature, taken out of the fridge at least 3 hours before using
- ½ tsp xanthan gum, or substitute with guar gum
- ¾ cup sugar substitute (xylitol, or monk fruit stevia blend, or erythritol)
- ¼ tsp ginger ground (optional, can be left out if you don't like ginger)
- 2 Tbsp lemon juice
- ½ cup melted coconut oil, warm but not hot (melted butter be substituted for the oil)
- ¾ cup fresh or frozen blueberries
- 1 tsp vanilla extract/essence
- ¼ cup almonds sliced for topping (optional)

Instructions

1. Preheat the oven to 350 F (180 C) and line a 9 x 5 inches loaf pan with parchment paper. Make sure the paper extends over the sides of the pan and grease or spray the parchment paper as this will prevent the loaf from sticking to the paper. Set it aside.
2. Add the eggs and sweetener to a mixing bowl and beat to combine for 30 seconds.
3. Add the coconut flour, almond flour, baking powder, xanthan gum, and ground ginger (if using) to a separate large mixing bowl and stir.
4. Pour the cooled down melted coconut oil, egg mixture, vanilla, and lemon juice onto the flour mixture. Use a wooden spoon and stir to evenly combine the ingredients.
5. Stir the fresh blueberries into the bread batter and pour the batter into the parchment-lined loaf pan.
6. Sprinkle the sliced almonds on top press down slightly on the almonds as this will make them stick to the bread.

7. Bake for 60 - 75 minutes. Remove the loaf pan after 20 minutes of baking time and lightly cover the pan with foil and return the bread to the oven to continue baking.

8. Check the bread after 60 minutes by inserting a skewer or blunt knife into the center of the bread. If the skewer or knife comes out with only a few crumbs sticking to it, or clan, then the bread is done. If it is not ready, then return the bread to the oven and continue baking. Check again after 10 minutes. If the bread is still not done, continue baking for 5 minutes.

9. Allow the bread to cool down for 30 minutes in the baking pan and then remove the loaf by pulling it out of the pan by holding on to the parchment paper.

10. Cool bread at least for 3 hours, or overnight before slicing. It is important not to be impatient as this bread may fall apart if sliced when not cooled down properly.

Notes

1. The bread can be stored in an airtight container at room temperature for up to 3 days.
2. If you want to freeze the bread, slice it and store it in an airtight freezer container. Slices can be defrosted at room temperature.

Vanilla Pound Cake Loaf (Gluten-Free)

Prep Time: 10 minutes

Cook Time: 50 minutes

Serving Size: Yields 12 slices, 1 slice per serving

Nutritional Facts/Info per serving:

Calories 170 Kcal
Carbs 3 g
Fat 14 g
Protein 7 g

Ingredients

- 2 cups almond flour
- 1 ½ tsp baking powder
- 2 Tbsp coconut flour
- 5 eggs, medium
- ¾ cup erythritol (see notes for brands)
- 3 Tbsp softened butter
- 3 Tbsp cream, heavy whipping
- ½ tsp lemon extract (optional)
- 1 tsp vanilla extract
- See notes for optional extras that can be added to the batter

Lemon Graze (Sugar-Free)

- 3 Tbsp lemon juice, fresh
- ½ cup Swerve Confectioners

Instructions

1. Preheat your oven to 350 F (180 C).
2. Spray a small loaf pan with vegetable oil, or grease it with butter. Then line the pan with parchment paper.

3. Place the butter, eggs, heavy cream, sweetener, lemon extract, and vanilla extract into a large mixing bowl. Use a hand mixer and whisk until the eggs are frothy about 2 - 3 minutes.
4. Put the coconut flour, baking powder, and almond flour into a separate mixing bowl and combine.
5. Add the dry ingredients to the bowl holding the wet ingredients and mix until all the ingredients are well combined.
6. Spoon the batter into the prepared loaf pan and use a spatula to smooth out the top.
7. Bake the loaf for 50 - 60 minutes. The loaf is done when a test skewer comes out clean.
8. Place the loaf on a cooling rack to cool down completely.
9. Make the lemon glaze by whisking the lemon juice and powdered sweetener together until you have a smooth glaze.
10. Drizzle the lemon glaze over the loaf only once it has cooled down completely.

Notes

1. This loaf is gluten-free, sugar-free, dairy-free, and grain-free.
2. Here are the top brands of erythritol available in the US as a guideline:
    a. Swerve.
    b. Pure Organic.
    c. Anthony's premium erythritol sweetener.
    d. Halefresh.
    e. NOW Foods.
    f. So Nourished.
    g. Hoosier Hills Farm.
    h. Whole Earth Sweetener Co.
3. The loaf can be stored in an airtight container at room temperature for 3 - 4 days. If you prefer to store it in the refrigerator, then reheat the slices in the microwave oven for a few seconds to soften them before serving.
4. The vanilla loaf is suitable for freezing, but it is recommended that the loaf is frozen without the glaze. Slice the loaf and use parchment paper to wrap the slices individually before freezing. Apply the glaze once you have defrosted and reheated the slices.

5. The following optional extras can be added to the loaf but it will make a slight difference to the nutritional values:
   a. Pecans.
   b. Chocolate chips, sugar-free.
   c. Walnuts.
   d. Cream cheese.
   e. Lemon zest.
   f. Cinnamon.
   g. Orange zest.

CHAPTER 8: PIZZA AND BREADSTICKS

This chapter provides a variety of pizza and breadsticks that will be loved by the whole family as main dishes and as snacks.

Creamy Mushroom Pizza

Prep Time: 15 minutes

Cook Time: 30 minutes

Serving Size: serves 4, ¼ of the pizza is one serving

Nutritional Facts/Info per serving:

Calories 467 Kcal
Carbs 7 g
Fat 38 g
Protein 19 g

Ingredients for Crust

- ⅞ cup (4 ½ oz) shredded zucchini
- ⅓ cup almond flour
- ½ cup shredded mozzarella cheese
- 1 egg, large
- 1 tsp salt
- ⅛ cup chia seeds
- ¼ cup water
- 3 Tbsp psyllium husk powder, ground

Ingredients for Topping

- ¼ cup cream cheese
- ¾ cup mozzarella cheese, shredded
- ¼ cup parmesan cheese, shredded
- ½ cup cream, heavy whipping
- 1 ¼ cup mushrooms, sliced
- 1 Tbsp butter, unsalted
- 3 minced garlic cloves
- 7 Tbsp scallions, sliced thinly
- 3 ⅔ Tbsp fresh parsley, minced
- ½ cup minced kale
- salt and pepper to taste

Instructions for Crust

1. Preheat the oven to 350 F (180 C).
2. Line a 15 x 10 inches baking pan or baking sheet with parchment paper.
3. Place all the pizza crust ingredients into a medium mixing bowl and combine. Once combined knead the mixture for a few minutes until it forms a firm dough.
4. Place the dough in the center of the parchment paper in the baking sheet and then place another sheet of parchment paper on top of the dough.
5. Use a rolling pin or your hands to flatten the dough and spread it across the pan to form a rectangular crust. Spread the dough evenly and remove some dough where the dough is thicker and place the pieces where the dough is thinner.
6. Pre-bake the crust for 15 minutes, the crust should be slightly golden brown. Remove from the oven and set aside to allow it to cool down.

Instructions for Topping

1. Prepare the mushroom topping while the crust is being pre-baked.
2. Place a large frying pan on the stove on medium. Add the butter and melt.
3. Sauté the mushrooms until it is slightly browned, about 5 minutes. Add the garlic and minced scallions and stir until it is translucent and tender. Reduce the heat to medium-low.
4. Pour the cream into the frying pan and then add the cream cheese. Keep stirring until the cheese is completely melted and the sauce has thickened slightly.
5. Add the parmesan cheese and kale and stir the mixture until well combined. Then remove the frying pan from the heat.
6. Spread the mushroom sauce mixture over the pizza crust evenly. Make sure to leave ¼ of the crust around the edges bare.
7. Sprinkle the parsley and mozzarella cheese over the sauce and season to taste with salt and pepper.
8. Place the pizza in the oven on the middle rack and bake until the mozzarella cheese is bubbly, about 15 minutes. Do not leave the pizza in the oven too long or it will brown too much and might burn. The pizza must be slightly golden brown.
9. Allow the pizza to cool down for a few minutes and then slice into 4 pieces and serve warm.

Notes

1. You can increase the protein by adding sliced ham, or prosciutto, or leftover cooked chicken. Remember to adjust your calories when any optional topping ingredients are added.

Cheesy Twists With Pesto

Prep Time: 10 minutes

Cook Time: 20 minutes

Serving Size: 10 cheesy twists, 1 twist per serving

Nutritional Facts/Info per serving:

Calories 181 Kcal
Carbs 1 g
Fat 16 g
Protein 7 g

Ingredients

- ¼ cup coconut flour
- ½ cup almond flour
- 1 tsp baking powder
- 1 beaten egg
- 2 ⅔ cups shredded mozzarella cheese
- butter
- ¼ cup green pesto
- 1 tsp baking powder
- ½ tsp salt
- 1 beaten egg for brushing the tops of the twists

Instructions

1. Preheat the oven to 350 F (180 C).
2. Prepare one flat baking pan 18 x 26 inches or two flat baking pans 13 x 18 inches. Cut two rectangular pieces of parchment paper the size of the large baking pan, or 4 sheets if using two smaller baking pans and set aside.
3. Place all the dry ingredients into a mixing bowl and stir. Then add 1 beaten egg and combine the mixture.
4. Put the cheese and butter into a saucepan and melt on low heat.

Stir while melting until the mixture is smooth.

5. Add the cheese mixture to the dry ingredients slowly and mix until the dough has firmed up.

6. Place the dough onto the rectangular piece of parchment paper, or if using smaller baking pans, divide the dough into two pieces and place on two sheets of parchment.

7. Roll out the dough to ⅕-inch thickness with a rolling pin. If the dough is sticky, then place the second piece of parchment paper on top of the dough to make rolling it out easier.

8. Spread the pesto evenly across the top of the dough and then cut into 10 1-inch strips. Twist the strips and place them on the parchment paper onto the baking pan. (See notes).

9. Bake until twists are golden brown, about 15 - 20 minutes.

10. Place twists on a cooling rack to cool down and serve slightly warm or cold.

Notes

1. If you experience problems twisting the dough, or if you want different shaped twists, then use a cookie cutter and out the shape you want and then place two dough shapes on top of each other, making a sandwich with the pesto being the filling. Remember to count the shapes and divide the number into 10 servings to keep your nutritional values correct.

2. If you are not big on pesto, simply substitute with your favorite herbs and spices. Cumin, chili, curry, and paprika works well, and herbs like basil, thyme, and oregano pair well with the bread twists.

3. A portion of the mozzarella cheese can be replaced by parmesan cheese for variety and a flavor boost.

Pizza Bites

Prep Time: 15 minutes

Cook Time: 20 minutes

Serving Size: 3o bites, 1 bite per serving

Nutritional Facts/Info per serving:

Calories 82 Kcal
Carbs 13 g
Fat 7 g
Protein 3.9 g

Ingredients

- 3 beaten eggs, large
- 16 oz cooked Italian sausage, drained and chopped
- ½ cup softened cream cheese
- 1 ⅓ cup mozzarella, shredded
- ⅓ cup coconut flour
- 1 tsp garlic, minced
- ½ tsp baking powder
- 1 tsp Italian seasoning

Instructions

1. Preheat the oven to 350 F (180 C).
2. Spray a flat baking pan with vegetable oil or grease it with butter and set aside.
3. Put the cream cheese and cooked and chopped sausage into a large mixing bowl and combine.
4. Add the rest of the ingredients to the mixing bowl and stir until well mixed.
5. Place the bowl of batter into the refrigerator for at least 10 minutes to chill. This allows the flour to absorb more of the liquid in the batter.

6. It is very important not to skip chilling the dough. The unchilled dough will flatten and spread when baked instead of forming round balls.
7. Use a cookie scoop to drop scoops of dough onto the prepared baking pan.
8. Bake until golden brown, about 18 - 2o minutes.
9. Cool the pizza bites down slightly and serve with a dipping sauce of your preference.

Notes

1. Experiment to see what size dough scoop gives you 30 pizza bites. or if you prefer bigger bites, then make 15 balls and each bite will then count as 2 servings.
2. 1 ½ cups of pepperoni chopped can be used instead of the Italian sausage.
3. Optional extras such as chopped mushrooms, black olives, and bell peppers can be added. Make sure that you pat dry whatever vegetables you add so that it does not add any liquid to the dough.
4. The pizza bites can be served cold and are ideal for lunch boxes as a snack.
5. The pizza bites can be frozen after baking for up to 3 months. Reheat in the microwave in increments of 20 seconds before serving.

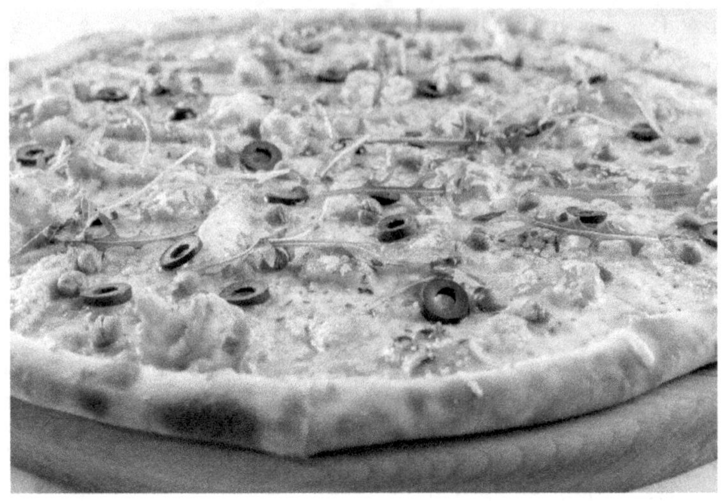

Gluten-Free Chicken Alfredo Pizza

Prep Time: 10 minutes

Cook Time: 35 minutes

Serving Size: 4 servings, ¼ of the pizza

Nutritional Facts/Info per serving:

Calories 329 Kcal
Carbs 8 g
Fat 23 g
Protein 21 g

Ingredients for Crust

- 3 Tbsp coconut flour
- 2 Tbsp golden flax, ground (can add extra almond flour instead)
- 3 Tbsp almond flour
- ¼ cup gluten-free alfredo sauce at room temperature
- 1 egg at room temperature
- 1 cup mozzarella cheese, shredded
- ¼ tsp garlic powder, roasted or regular

Ingredients for Topping

- 1 small oz can of chicken breast, drain the liquid off
- ½ cup mozzarella cheese, shredded
- ½ gluten-free alfredo sauce
- ½ tsp garlic powder, regular or roasted

Instructions

1. Preheat the oven to 425 F (220 C).
2. Place all the crust ingredients, except the mozzarella cheese, in the bowl of a food processor.
3. Place 1 cup of mozzarella cheese in a microwave-safe bowl and melt the cheese until completely melted, stirring every 30 seconds.
4. Add the melted cheese to the dry ingredients and mix using the dough blade until all the ingredients are fully combined and the dough has a consistent color.
5. Spread the dough on a pizza stone, a pizza pan, or an inverted flat baking pan and place it on the bottom rack in the oven. Bake until the crust is golden brown, about 20 minutes.
6. While the crust is baking, mix the chicken, garlic powder, and alfredo sauce in a mixing bowl and set aside.
7. Remove the pizza crust from the oven and reduce the heat to 350 F (180 C).
8. Top the crust with the chicken alfredo mixture and sprinkle the mozzarella cheese on top.
9. Place the pizza in the oven on the top rack and bake for a further 15 minutes. The pizza is ready when the cheese starts to bubble.
10. Remove from the oven and cut into 4 equal-sized slices and serve.

Notes

1. Optional extras suggested are below. Vegetables will not affect your nutritional values much, but extra carbs and protein will, so please keep that in mind.
   a. Bacon.
   b. Blue cheese.
   c. Broccoli.
   d. Bell peppers.
   e. Spinach.
   f. Fresh parsley.
   g. Fresh cilantro.
2. You can store any leftover pizza in the fridge for up to 4 days. Reheat pizza in the oven on low heat in a covered dish or skillet. You can reheat it in the microwave, but it will lose the crispness of the crust.

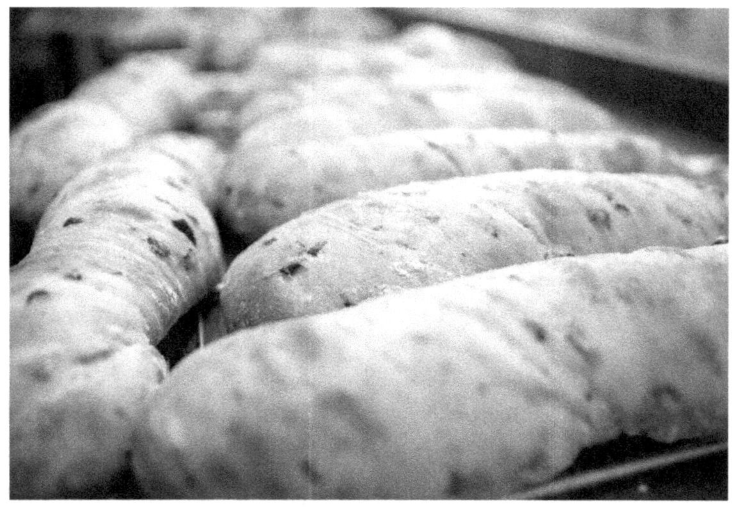

Gluten-Free Italian Breadsticks

Prep Time: 20 minutes + 30 minutes chill time

Cook Time: 22 minutes

Serving Size: 8 breadsticks, 1 per serving

Nutritional Facts/Info per serving:

Calories 302 Kcal
Carbs 6 g
Fat 24 g
Protein 15 g

Ingredients *for Dough*

- 3 cups of grated mozzarella cheese
- 2 eggs, large, and whisked
- ¼ cup cubed cream cheese
- 1 ¾ cups almond flour
- 1 Tbsp baking powder
- 2 tsp garlic powder

Ingredients *for Topping*

- 2 tsp Italian seasoning
- 2 Tbsp melted butter
- 2 tsp salt

Instructions

1. Preheat the oven to 350 F (180 C).
2. Line a flat baking pan with parchment paper and set it aside.
3. Place the shredded mozzarella and cream cheese in a microwave-safe bowl for 90 seconds. Stir halfway through so that the cheese melts evenly.
4. Add the almond flour, beaten egg, baking powder, and garlic powder to the cheese mixture and mix until dough forms, making sure the ingredients are fully combined.
5. Place the dough into the refrigerator for 30 minutes to chill. This step is needed as it makes the dough less sticky and firms up the dough.
6. Cut the dough into 8 equal pieces. Oil your hands and then roll each piece into a tube about 1 inch thick and 6 inches long and place breadsticks onto the baking pan. Use a pastry brush and brush the melted butter over the tops and then sprinkle the salt and Italian seasoning over.
7. Bake until breadsticks are golden, for about 18 - 20 minutes.
8. Serve with a dipping sauce of your own preference.

Notes

1. The breadsticks can be stored in an airtight container on a countertop for a few days, but be aware that they will lose their very crispy crust. Breadsticks are always best to be eaten on the day of baking.
2. Do not freeze the raw breadsticks dough as any dough that contains cream cheese will be watery when defrosted.

CHAPTER 9:
FUN KETO BREAD FOR THE WHOLE FAMILY

Keto bread does not only mean standard loaf bread. Here is a selection of fun types of bread that the whole family will enjoy, as well as being a great hit with guests.

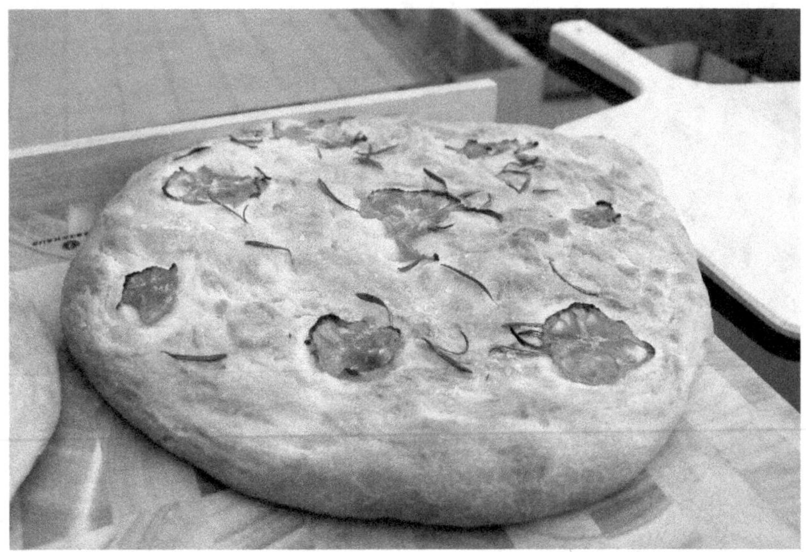

Rosemary and Garlic Focaccia Bread

Prep Time: 10 minutes

Cook Time: 20 minutes

Serving Size: 8 slices, 1 slice per serving (2 half slices)

Nutritional Facts/Info per serving:

Calories 196 Kcal
Carbs 3 g
Fat 17 g
Protein 8 g

Ingredients for Dough

- ¾ cup almond flour
- 1 ½ cups shredded mozzarella cheese
- 2 tsp erythritol, optional (see notes)
- 2 Tbsp cream cheese
- 1 egg
- ½ tsp salt
- ½ tsp garlic powder
- 1 tsp vinegar, white wine
- black olives, pitted and sliced, optional
- love, not optional

Ingredients Butter Topping

- 1 tsp powdered garlic or finely chopped fresh garlic
- ¼ cup butter at room temperature
- 2 tsp finely chopped fresh rosemary or 1 tsp dried rosemary
- ½ tsp salt

Instructions

1. Preheat the oven to 400 F (200 C).
2. Place the cream cheese and mozzarella cheese in a large microwave-safe bowl and melt the cheese for about 90 seconds, stirring every 30 seconds. Be careful not to burn the cheese and remove the bowl as soon as the cheese has melted.
3. Add all the other dough ingredients to the cheese and mix to combine.
4. Shape the dough into an 8-inch round flat disk and place it on a piece of parchment paper and then into a flat baking pan.
5. Poke holes into the focaccia dough several times.
6. Place in the oven and bake until the bread is golden brown, about 12 minutes.
7. Remove from the oven and allow the bread to cool down slightly so that you can handle it.

8. Make the butter topping while the bread is baking by mixing the garlic, butter, rosemary, and salt in a small bowl.
9. Spread the butter mixture over the top of the bread and return it to the oven to bake for an extra 8 - 10 minutes. Check regularly and if the focaccia is a deep brown, remove it from the oven.
10. Divide the focaccia into 8 slices and serve warm.

Notes

1. Focaccia can be stored at room temperature for up to 2 days if covered with plastic wrap and for up to 4 days in the fridge placed in an airtight plastic bag.
2. It can be frozen for up to 1 month as individual slices using resealable plastic bags.
3. Reheat leftover focaccia in the oven for 10 minutes at 375 F (190 C) or place it in a toaster oven and drizzle a small amount of oil over the top.

Gluten-Free Flatbread

Prep Time: 10 minutes

Cook Time: 15 minutes

Serving Size: 1 flatbread 8 slices, 1 slice per serving

Nutritional Facts/Info per serving:

Calories 151 Kcal
Carbs 2 g
Fat 12 g
Protein 9 g

Ingredients

- ½ cup almond flour
- 2 Tbsp cream cheese
- 2 cups shredded mozzarella cheese
- 2 eggs, well beaten
- salt and pepper to taste
- 1 - 2 tsp of spice and herb mixture of your choice (optional)

Instructions

1. Preheat the oven to 350 F (180 C),
2. Line one or two flat baking pans with parchment paper and set them aside.
3. Put the mozzarella and cream cheese into a large microwave-proof dish and mix. Melt the cheese in increments of 30 seconds and stir each time until the cheese is melted and has no lumps.
4. Place the flour, salt and pepper, and egg into a large mixing bowl and mix. Add half of the cheese mixture to the flour mixture and stir. Repeat with the second half of the cheese mixture.
5. Once the dough holds together transfer it to the baking pan and flatten the dough evenly in the pan.

6. You can make 8 individual round flatbreads by dividing the dough into 8 equal portions. Make balls and place four balls on each of the two baking pans. Flatten the dough to form round flatbread.
7. Sprinkle any additional optional seasonings over the top of the flatbread.
8. Bake until the bread is golden brown, about 15 - 17 minutes.
9. Place the flatbread on a cooling rack to cool down before serving.

Notes

1. Carbalose flour can be substituted for almond flour on a 1:1 basis.
2. It is best to always store flatbread in an airtight container in the refrigerator for up to 5 days.
3. Flatbread can be frozen for up to 2 months. Place individual servings in separate resealable freezer bags.
4. Reheat the flatbread by wrapping it in a damp kitchen towel and placing it on a plate in the microwave for about 30 seconds.
5. This flatbread is suitable to be used for sandwiches, as a pizza base, or as a wrap.

Bread Rolls

Prep Time: 20 minutes

Cook Time: 13 - 18 minutes

Serving Size: 12 rolls, 1 roll per serving

Nutritional Facts/Info per serving:

Calories 261 Kcal
Carbs 4.2 g
Fat 20.5 g

Protein 14.4 g

Ingredients

- 2 ¼ cups almond flour
- ¼ cup coconut flour
- 3 cups mozzarella cheese, shredded
- ½ cup cream cheese, full fat
- 2 eggs
- 1 egg for egg wash (see notes)
- ½ cup buttermilk or low carb yogurt, plain
- ½ tsp baking soda
- ½ tsp baking powder
- ½ tsp salt

Instructions

1. Preheat the oven to 400 F (200 C).
2. Line a flat baking pan with parchment paper and set it aside.
3. Place the cream cheese and mozzarella cheese in a glass bowl and microwave until the cheese has melted, stirring every 30 seconds. Alternatively, you can use a non-stick skillet and melt the cheese on the stovetop, stirring frequently until the cheese has melted fully.

4. Add all the remaining ingredients to the food processor bowl and then add the melted cheese. Pulse until the mixture is well mixed. You can also do this with an electric mixer but it will take longer for the dough to come together.
5. Work with the dough by either wetting your hands or drizzling some oil on your hands. This helps greatly to stop the dough from sticking to your hands while forming dough balls.
6. Make 12 dough balls of even size and place them on the parchment-lined baking pan. Make sure that there is at least 1-inch space between each roll.
7. Place the last egg into a small bowl and whisk well. Brush egg wash over the rolls.
8. Bake in the center of the oven for 13 - 18 minutes. The rolls are done when the outside has hardened and feels slightly firm to the touch, and the rolls are golden brown.
9. Allow rolls to cool down for a few minutes before serving. These rolls are best eaten warm.

Notes

1. Always serve these rolls warm because when they cool down the rolls become hard and the cheese condenses.
2. The egg wash is optional. You can also brush the rolls with melted butter before baking.
3. The buttermilk can be substituted with sour cream.
4. Reheat leftover rolls in the microwave, oven, or toaster oven.
5. These rolls are not suitable for freezing.

Cheesy Bread Fingers

Prep Time: 10 minutes

Cook Time: 17 minutes

Serving Size: 8, 1 bread finger per serving (2 half bread fingers)

Nutritional Facts/Info per serving:

Calories 299 Kcal
Carbs 4 g
Fat 23 g
Protein 17 g

Ingredients for Bread Fingers

- ⅓ cup coconut flour
- 1 ½ cups mozzarella cheese
- 2 Tbsp cream cheese, softened
- ½ cup grated parmesan cheese
- 4 ½ Tbsp melted butter, cooled down
- 4 eggs
- ¼ tsp baking powder
- ¼ tsp salt
- ½ tsp garlic powder
- 1 tsp Italian seasoning

Ingredients for Topping

- ¼ cup grated parmesan cheese
- 2 cups shredded mozzarella cheese
- ½ tsp Italian seasoning

Instructions

1. Preheat the oven to 400 F (200 C).
2. Grease an 11 x 7 inches deep baking pan with butter or spray with vegetable spray.
3. Place the melted butter, salt, eggs, and cream cheese in a large mixing bowl and whisk until combined.
4. Add the baking powder, coconut flour, spices, and baking powder and stir until the mixture is well combined.
5. Stir in the parmesan and mozzarella cheese and pour the batter into the baking pan.
6. Top the bread batter with the topping ingredients.
7. Bake for 15 minutes.
8. Remove the bread halfway through the baking time and cut horizontally down the middle and vertically to create 16 half bread fingers.
9. Return the bread to the oven and continue baking until done.
10. Move the baking pan to the top rack and switch to broil until the cheese is bubbly and browned about 1 - 2 minutes.
11. Serve with a low-carb marinara sauce or dipping sauce of your choice.

Notes

1. You can use a rectangular casserole dish in place of the baking pan.
2. The bread fingers can be kept in the fridge for several days.
3. The bread fingers are suitable for freezing. Make sure that they are completely cooled down before putting them into the freezer in a sealable freezer container or into individual servings in freezer bags.

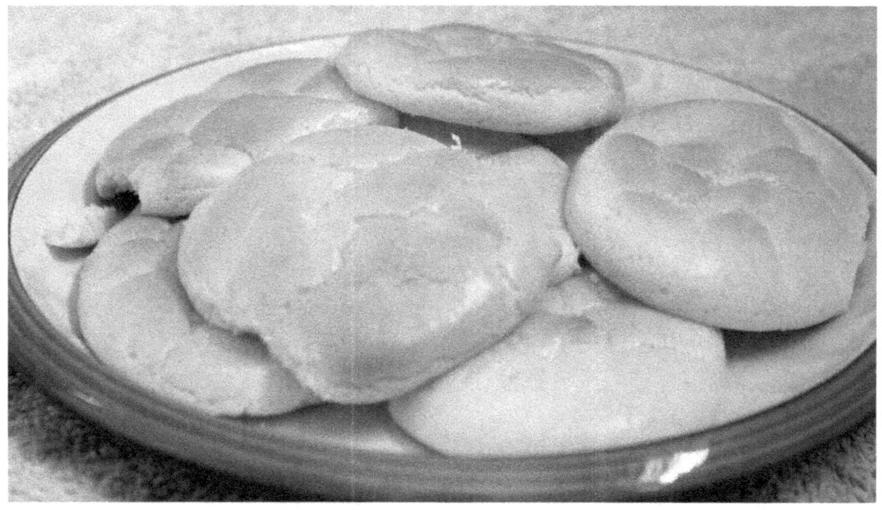

Cloud Bread (Gluten-Free)

Prep Time: 10 minutes

Cook Time: 30 minutes (15 minutes in a convection oven)

Serving Size: 10 pieces, 1 piece per serving

Nutritional Facts/Info per serving:

Calories 36 Kcal
Carbs 1 g
Fat 2 g
Protein 2 gram

Ingredients

- 4 eggs, yolks, and whites separated
- ¼ cup cream cheese, low-fat
- ½ tsp cream of tartar
- ¼ - ½ tsp garlic powder
- 1 tsp Italian seasoning
- ½ tsp salt

Instructions

1. Preheat the oven to 300 F (150 C).
2. Line two large flat baking pans with parchment paper and set them aside.
3. Separate the egg whites and yolks.
4. Put the egg whites into a stand mixer and then add the cream of tartar. Use the whip attachment of the mixer and beat on high until the mixture forms stiff meringue peaks. Scrape the meringue out into a mixing bowl.
5. Put the cream cheese into the bowl of the stand mixer and beat to soften the cheese on high.
6. Add the egg yolks to the cheese one at a time. Beat until the mixture is smooth and egg yolks and cheese are fully incorporated. Scrape the sides of the bowl to ensure that ingredients blend well.
7. Add the salt, garlic powder, and Italian seasoning and beat again.
8. Fold the meringue into the egg mixture very gently using a spatula. It is important to deflate the meringue as little as possible. The mixture must be foamy and firm.
9. Use a ¼ cup measure to spoon the mixture onto the baking pans leaving enough space between the foam portions to be able to spread each foam portion out. Spread each foam portion into 4-inch circles about ¾-inch high.
10. Bake the cloud bread until it is firm and golden on the outside.30 minus in a normal oven and about 15 - 18 minutes in a convection oven. The centers of the cloud bread should be firm enough so that it does not jiggle if you shake it.
11. Leave the cloud bread on the baking pan to cool down as freshly baked cloud bread can be fragile.
12. Once cooled down, remove from the baking pan and serve.

Notes

1. The texture of cloud bread is at its best in the first 12 hours after baking but can be stored in the fridge for up to 5 days in an airtight container.
2. Cloud bread is very versatile and can be used in many ways.
    a. Plain as a snack.
    b. Sandwiches.
    c. Burgers.
    d. Sliders.
    e. Pizza bases.
    f. Eat with soup.

CONCLUSION

The ketogenic diet is a healthy alternative to the typical westernized diet we're used to. It's relatively simple to understand and implement. The health benefits are numerous and, unlike conventional diets, you don't have to half-starve yourself to see results. Teaching your body to burn fat for fuel instead of carbs helps to kick start the burning of excess body fat in the process. This makes it easier and more effective to lose weight, get healthy, and feel great.

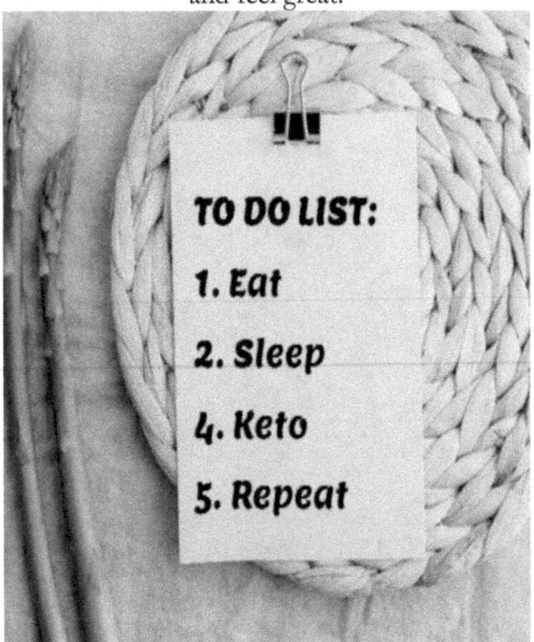

Everyone can successfully follow the keto diet; from athletes to the average person working in an office. The best part is you don't have to deprive yourself of your favorite foods either. Take bread, for example, we've just shown you that bread can fit into your keto diet without ruining your progress or derailing your body's ketosis. These tasty recipes are great for all sorts of occasions and for sharing with friends and family. Never feel left out again when those close to you are enjoying carb-laden bread while you watch on, unable to join in. Now you can make tasty bread that everyone will love and you can enjoy it too without an ounce of guilt.

Use our great-tasting recipes to tantalize your taste buds by baking your bread in the comfort of your kitchen. It's simple, it's easy, it's nutritious, and it's delicious to make your own bread. It's even easier if you have a bread machine handy that will do most of the work for you.

125

You have the knowledge and the recipes; all you have to do is buy the ingredients.

What are you waiting for?

Get baking today and you will never miss traditional bread again.

Thank you for choosing this book, I hope you got something away from it, even if just a full belly. If you did, I would be delighted to receive your honest review. Enjoy your meal, family and life without regrets.

-Paul

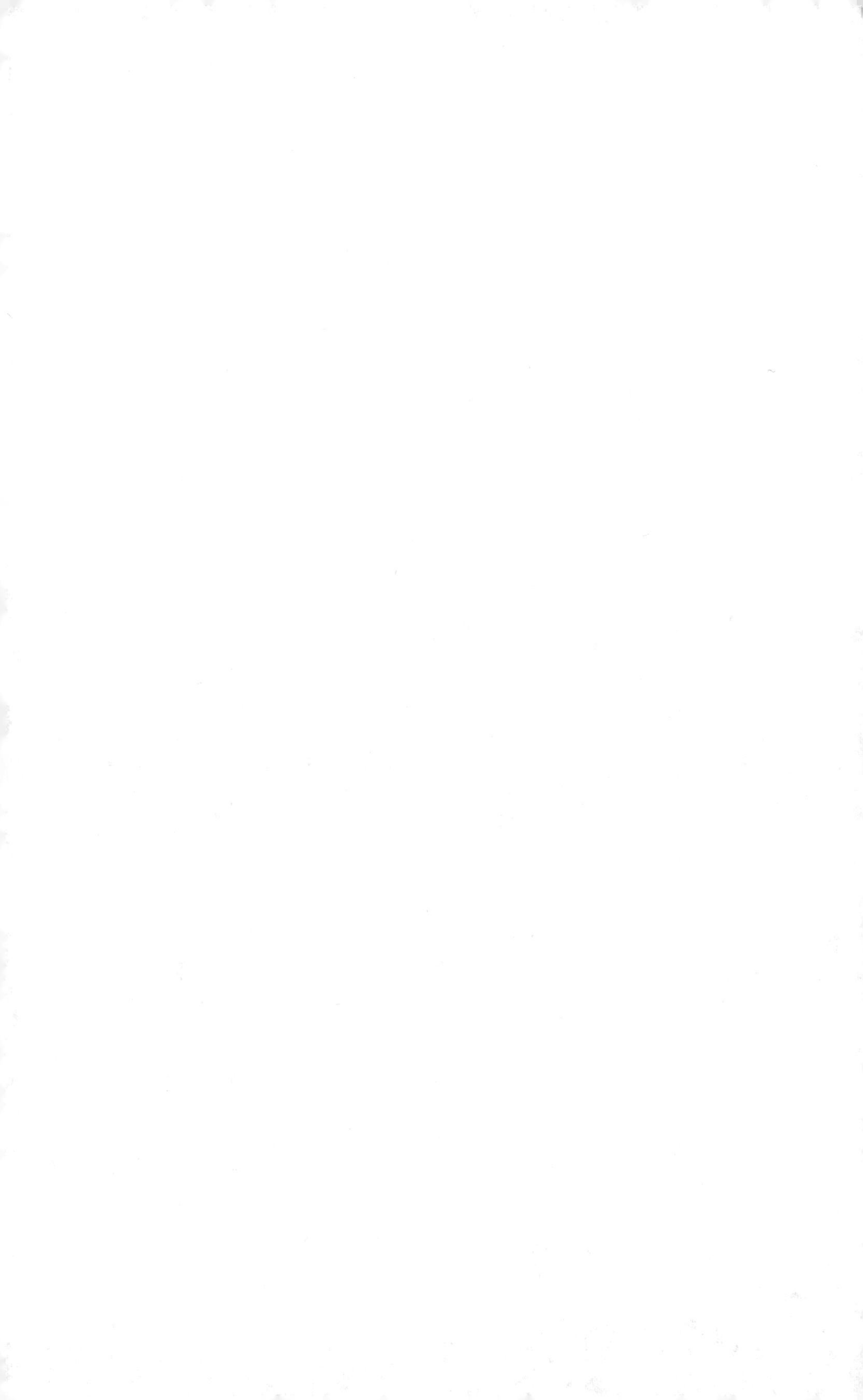